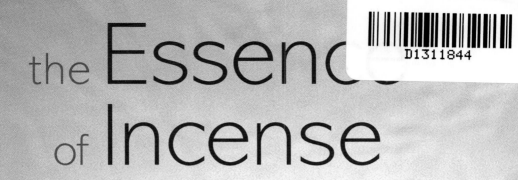

the Essence of Incense

Bringing Fragrance into the Home

DIANA ROSEN

Photographs by Giles D. Prett

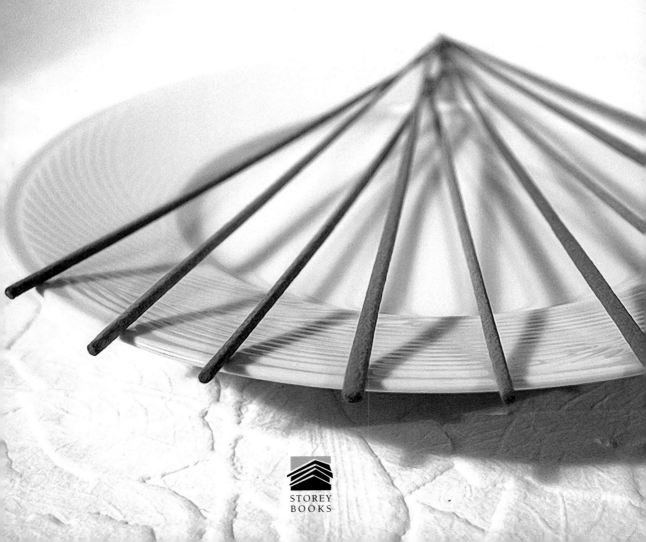

STOREY BOOKS

The mission of Storey Communications is to serve our customers by publishing practical information that encourages personal independence in harmony with the environment.

Edited by Deborah Balmuth and Larry Shea
Cover design by Mark Tomasi
Cover photograph by Giles Prett
Photographs by Giles Prett/SCI, except for photo on page 66 by Cynthia McFarland
Photo styling by Mark Tomasi, Cynthia McFarland, and Giles Prett
Book design and production by Mark Tomasi
Art direction by Cynthia McFarland
Indexed by Deborah Burns
Thanks to Anna's Incense, Hope, B.C., Canada; Avid Inc., New Paltz, NY; The Cottage, Williamstown, MA; Paula Walla Imports, Windsor Locks, CT; Pier 1 Imports, Pittsfield, MA; Sarut NYC, New York, NY; and Shoyeido Corp., Boulder, CO, for the use of props.

Storey Books are available for special premium and promotional uses and for customized editions. For further information, call Storey's Custom Publishing Department at 1-800-793-9396.

Printed in Canada by Transcontinental Printing
10 9 8 7 6 5 4 3 2 1

Library of Congress Cataloging-in-Publication Data

Rosen, Diana.
    The essence of incense: bringing fragrance into the home/by Diana Rosen.
        p. cm.
    ISBN 1-58017-367-5 (alk. paper)
    1. Aromatherapy. I. Title.

RM666.A68 R674 2001
615'.321--dc21   2001020766

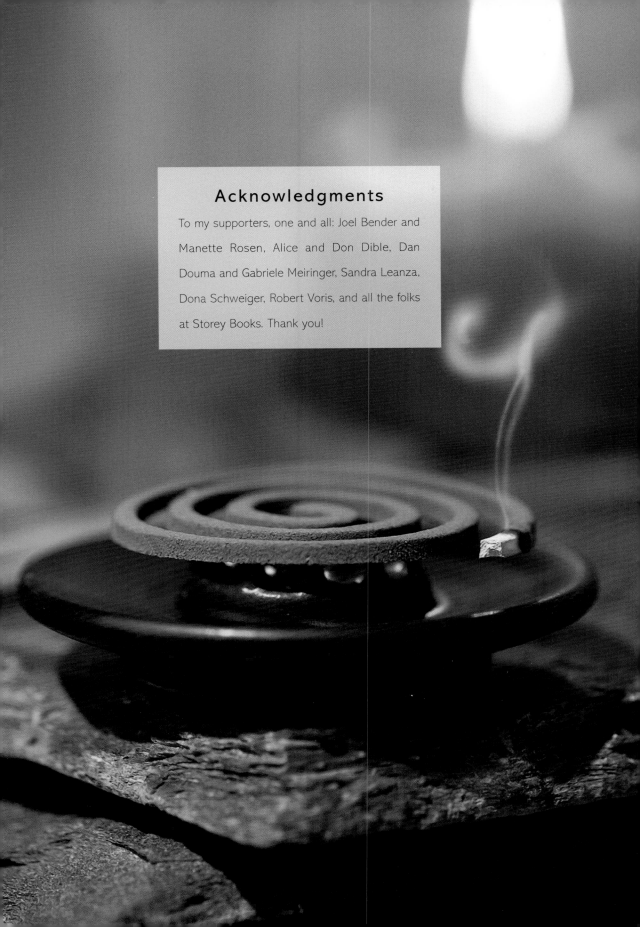

Acknowledgments

To my supporters, one and all: Joel Bender and Manette Rosen, Alice and Don Dible, Dan Douma and Gabriele Meiringer, Sandra Leanza, Dona Schweiger, Robert Voris, and all the folks at Storey Books. Thank you!

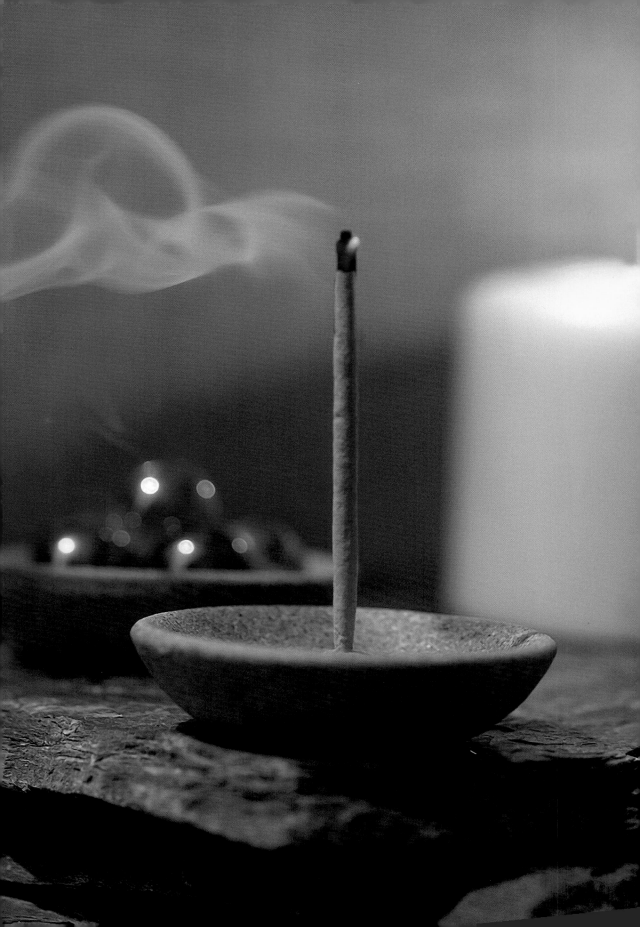

contents

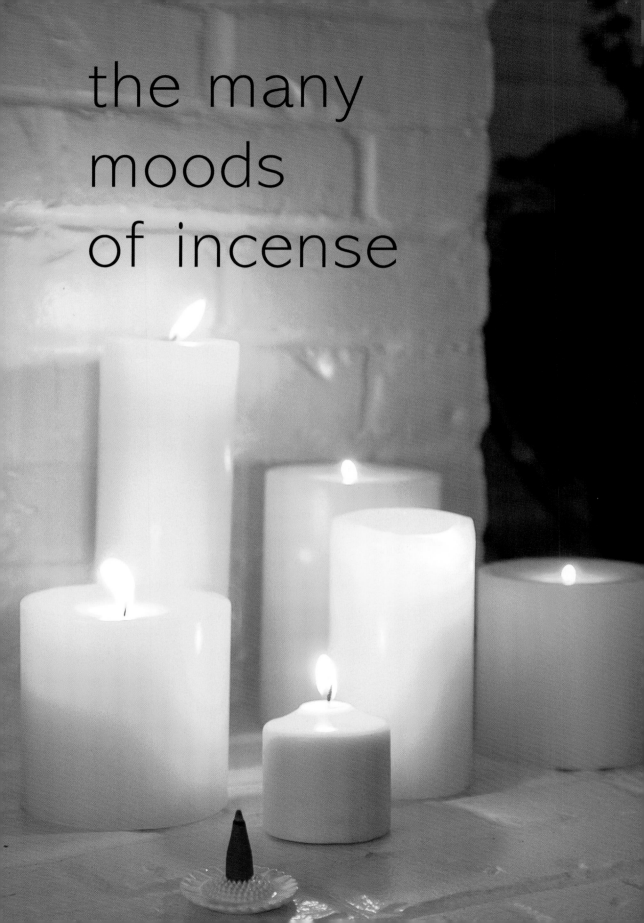

the many
moods
of incense

ncense is the ultimate home fragrance. It does more than simply make our surroundings smell better. Like other forms of aromatherapy, carefully chosen incense can have the effect of de-stressing, energizing, or relaxing those who inhale its smoke. Moreover, the evocative scents of frankincense, lavender, cinnamon, jasmine, juniper, or cloves encourage us to slow down, stop the busyness, and become mindful of the present moment.

Perhaps the most powerful element of incense is its ability to draw us into meditative states from which we can gather clarity, strength, and motivation to pursue our daily lives. It offers a tool for reaching deeper inside ourselves to gain personal understanding and greater awareness of the world around us.

As you experiment and explore the many incense fragrances available today, you will discover that any activity can be enhanced by "listening to incense," as the Chinese and Japanese describe the burning of fragrance sticks. As aromatherapists have discovered, scent has the ability to change a mood, highlight an experience, add an extra dimension to anything you already do, or just create an inviting ambience.

The ancient Chinese believed that different scents induced different reactions: tranquility, reclusivity (peaceful solitude), luxury, beauty, refinement, and even nobility. *Heang,* the words used for the pleasure and benefits of aromas, formed a whole concerto of fragrant notes in the Chinese vocabulary. We might choose other words than nobility or luxury to describe how scent affects us, but we now know that odors have a powerful effect upon people. In this book, I offer suggestions for using incense to create moods in your home, enhance common activities, and set the scene for meaningful, reflective moments, both alone and shared with those you love and live with.

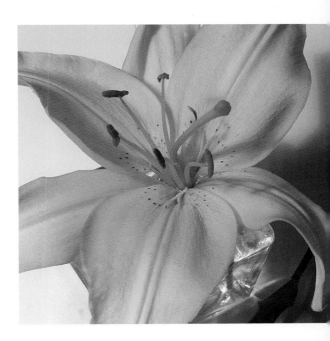

Three things revive a person's soul: pleasant sights, pleasant sounds, and pleasant smells.

The Talmud

Incense Every Day

While burning incense is appropriate for marking special occasions, it is also suitable for daily use. Think about how your daily chores might be enhanced with just a touch of fragrance in the air. As you iron, for example, try misting your clothes with rosemary water before applying the warm iron, or set a joss stick of incense in a censer nearby to waft around you.

You might then experience ironing as a pleasurable experience rather than just a task to get through. Reflect on the associations of the piece you are ironing. Damask tablecloths or heirloom bed linens can remind you of all those people who enjoyed these fine fabrics before you, whether they were family or the strangers who had them before they fell from grace to the flea market where you bought them. Focus on appreciating the simple act of ironing and its immediate satisfactions: A smooth stroke of the cloth and all the wrinkles are erased.

Other chores such as polishing silver or brass candlesticks or plates are brightened and made special when the scent of clove incense surrounds you. Witness the dance of your hands as they move the polishing cloth about, and observe the reflection of your contented face in the shining mirror of metal.

The sweet scent of vanilla will enhance time spent quietly sewing, knitting, or doing home repairs such as caulking a bathtub or repairing a loose doorknob. The fragrance relaxes your body, enabling your hands to pursue these everyday tasks with a rhythm that maks them more successful and enjoyable. All of these ordinary gestures can become meditations for the soul when you "listen to incense."

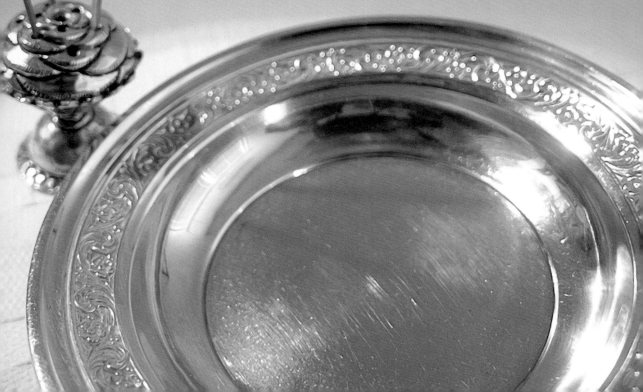

Selecting
Incense Fragrances

Let your nose lead you to what intrigues, fascinates, or pleases you. The only requirement is that the fragrance should be a welcoming addition, not an intrusion. You might turn to aromatherapy for an understanding of the effects of various scents. For example, the biting effervescence of an orange is considered an uplifting and energizing scent; the sweetness of the tiny violet is sleep-inducing; and the smoky softness of frankincense and myrrh is peaceful. Experiment to see how different fragrances affect you. Try gardenias or roses, rosemary or sage, or any of the hundreds of other incense fragrances available.

Experiment with styles of incense, too: Choose a coil one time and loose powder the next; a simple stick this morning and perhaps copal and charcoal this evening. Incense is economical; you can try a new type every day for a week and spend barely five dollars.

Eventually, you may develop a signature scent, just as perfume makers create personalized perfumes or essences. Sample different brands of your favorite scent to see which one pleases you, or make a combination of two or three that signal your personality. Light your signature incense in your home just before people come to call. They'll instantly be transported to the right mood of remembering other happy times you've spent together.

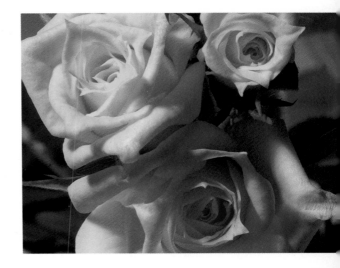

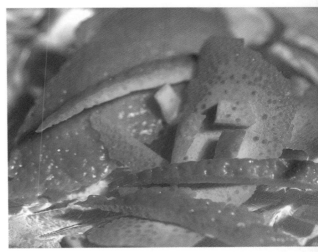

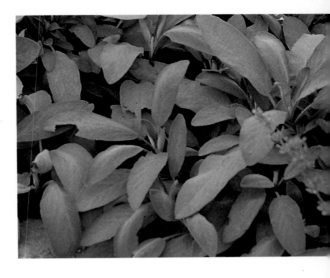

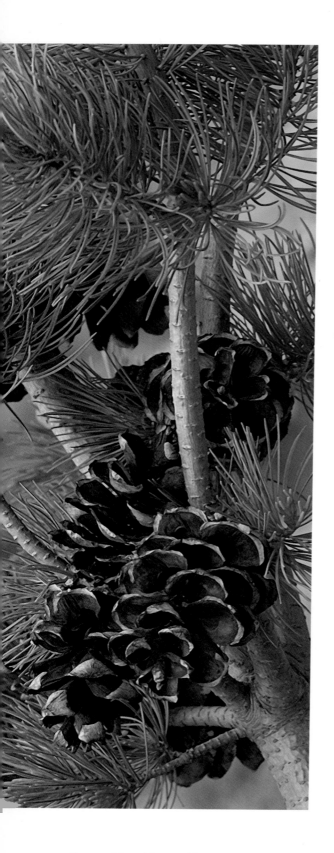

Fragrance Families

Today's great selection of incense reflects scent memories like the homey smells of freshly mowed grass, fresh-baked bread, or just-laundered sheets drying in the noonday sun.

Woodsy scents tend to transport one to calmness. Such earthy scents include cedar, meditative aloeswood (also called agarwood or oud), energizing pine, therapeutic camphor, sensuous sandal-wood, and any resinous tree like frankin-cense or myrrh.

Floral fragrances attach most vividly to sense memory. Sweeter fra-grances are more likely to induce sleep, like violets, or to be sensuous, like jas-mine. Rose, gardenia, or orange blossoms are stimulating to our sexual energy. Other classic flowers used for incense include lilac, lilies, honeysuckle, white lotus, gera-nium, tuberose, and Indian kewra.

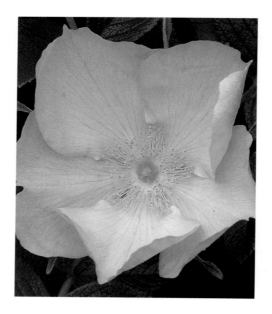

Fruity scents are uplifting and mood enhancing. Both traditional and contemporary incense have fruit-based fragrances, including berries, melons, bananas, kiwi, coconut, plum, apricot, and peach. Juniper berries, though poisonous if eaten, make a relaxing and sensuous incense.

Citrus fruit scents tend to be energizing and refreshing, doing much to restore confidence. Some choices commonly used in incense are: bergamot, neroli, mandarin, orange, grapefruit, lemon, and lime. Citronella, a grass, emits a wonderful citrusy scent and repels moths. Lemongrass, also a grass, is another popular citrusy scent.

Herbal and vegetative scents offer slightly herbaceous, even sweetly woodsy scents. Sweetgrass is indeed sweet and smells much like vanilla.

Savory spices and herbs like clove, cardamom, cassia, cinnamon, rosemary, and thyme offer clarity, stimulation, and energy. Other examples of stimulating spices and herbs are black pepper, aniseed, mustard, ginger, bay leaf, marjoram, oregano, coriander, turmeric, asafetida, and spearmint.

Note: Some herbs should be used with caution. Peppermint smells foul when burned; nutmeg is toxic in large doses; sage, thyme, rosemary, hyssop, and cedar may elevate blood pressure.

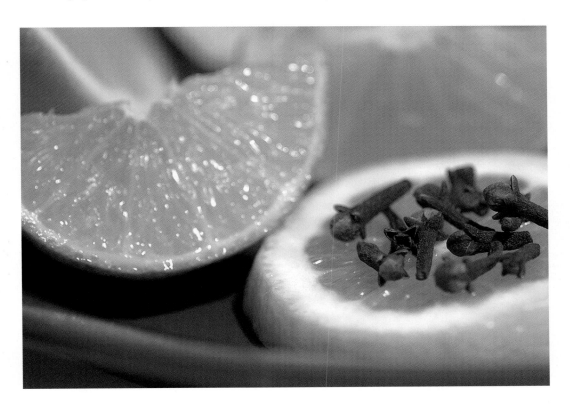

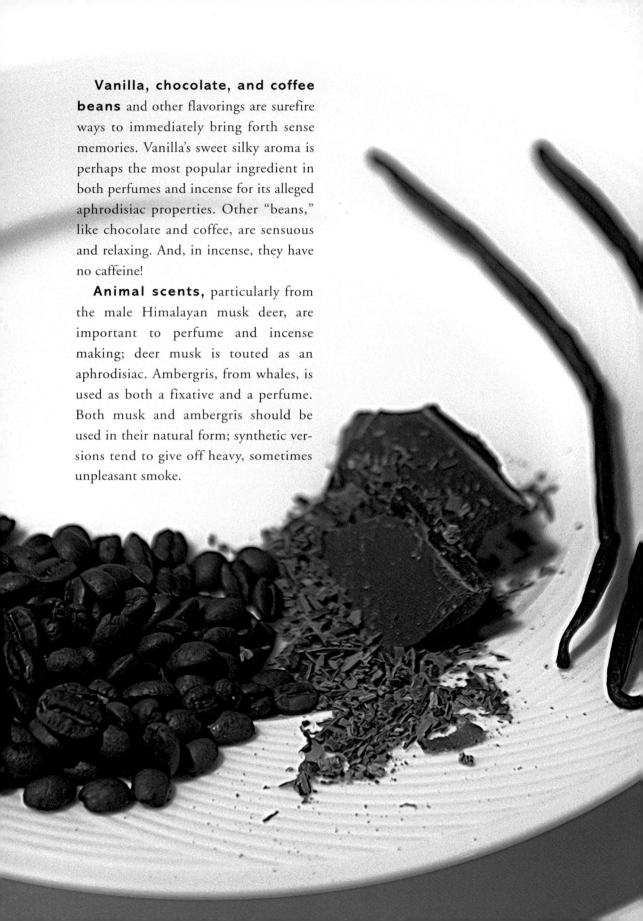

Vanilla, chocolate, and coffee beans and other flavorings are surefire ways to immediately bring forth sense memories. Vanilla's sweet silky aroma is perhaps the most popular ingredient in both perfumes and incense for its alleged aphrodisiac properties. Other "beans," like chocolate and coffee, are sensuous and relaxing. And, in incense, they have no caffeine!

Animal scents, particularly from the male Himalayan musk deer, are important to perfume and incense making; deer musk is touted as an aphrodisiac. Ambergris, from whales, is used as both a fixative and a perfume. Both musk and ambergris should be used in their natural form; synthetic versions tend to give off heavy, sometimes unpleasant smoke.

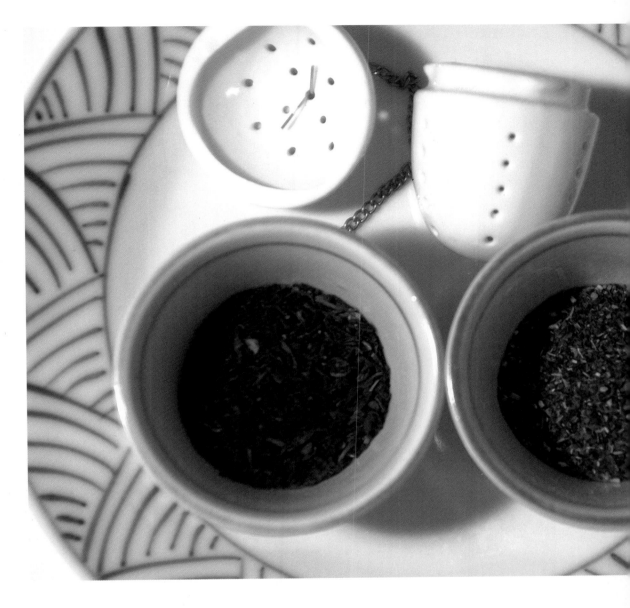

Tea is a new favorite for contemporary incense — Chinese and Japanese green teas for their sweet grassy aroma, Lapsang souchong and Yunnan for their smokiness, and Darjeeling and other fine blacks for their tangy sharpness. Classic scented teas are also used in incense: Earl Grey for its bergamot or lavender; Ceylon or Assam blacks with heavy fruit essences like blackberry, citrus, mandarin, or cherry.

An important note: If you are planning to make your own incense from any of these categories (see page 118 for directions), always burn some of the plant or herb by itself first. Some become noxious or unpleasant when burned and should not be used in incense.

Ancient Traditions

It is most likely that with the discovery of fire, scraps of resinous wood were tossed upon the flames, causing a remarkable fragrance to climb up among a mystic smoke. Around the campfire, shoulders relaxed, voices softened, all was calm and safe. Mankind had discovered the power of fragrant smoke, or incense.

As the human story progressed, so did our enchantment with fragrance. Herbs, grasses, spices, flowers, plants, and the bark and resins of many trees found their way into the practice of incense burning. The very word "perfume" comes from the Latin *per fumus,* through smoke.

The ancient Hebrews embraced cinnamon, rose, and cedar; frankincense and myrrh, aloeswood, and amber. Fabled sources of incense included the cedars of Lebanon, the kyphi flower, and the roses of Sharon. Across the ancient world, incense was burned and perfumed oils anointed body and clothing.

Incense has long been a traditional part of nearly every culture. For example, in many Chinese homes, the oldest woman in the family carries a stick of incense outside every morning, bows once to the god of heaven, once to the god of earth, and then re-enters her home. At the family altar, she bows a third time for the memory of all her ancestors. This custom will be passed on to her daughter-in-law, who will pass it on to her son's wife, as generations of women have done before them.

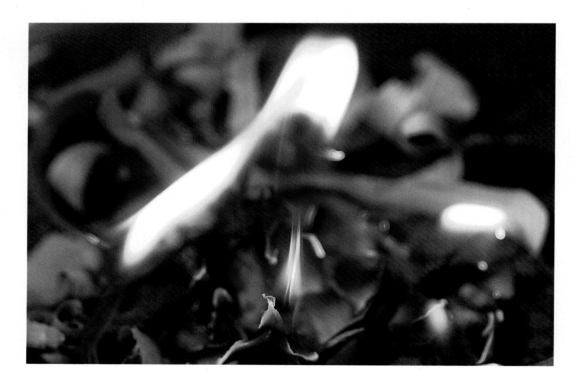

Incense and Memory

I remember when I first met him. It was in Washington, D.C., and the Japanese cherry blossoms were in bloom. It was a serendipitous summer of experiences when every adventure seemed imbued with magic. The object of my affection has long been gone from my life, but whenever nostalgia washes over me, I light some cherry incense and the happiness of that teenage summer becomes a living memory I can rerun in my mind once more.

Scent is like that. It triggers memories when you least expect it and transports you back to the past in the gentlest of ways. These smells might carry you to your favorite travel destinations: adventures up the Nile, sailing to tropical isles, or family trips to the mountains, where you ate fresh trout for breakfast.

Scent can remind you of other pleasures: the heady sugary smell of cotton candy at the county fair, or the tang of yeast as you walk by your neighborhood Italian bakery. Or perhaps the dank chill deep in a forest, or the crisp scent of paper as you open a brand-new book.

All these memories, and so many more, are part of the scrapbook of happy times you can experience through the power of incense. Lighting a peach-scented incense stick can take you to the afternoon when you ate the first freshly picked peaches of the season. A cone of pine or pinion incense can bring back a walk through the woods the first time you went away to camp.

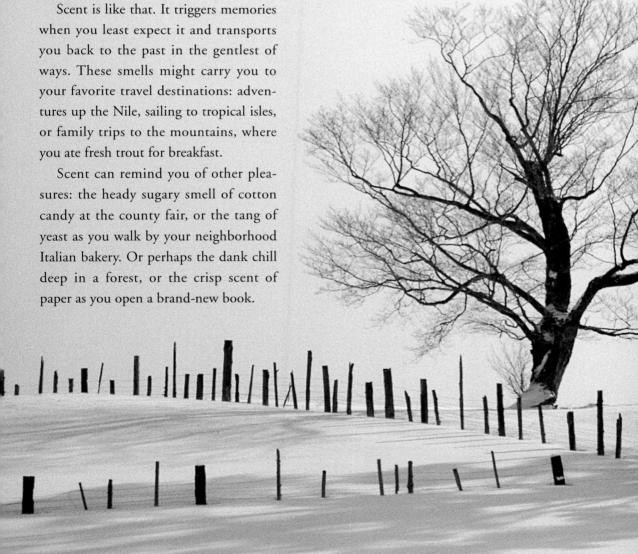

Just as scent can trigger memories of the past, it can create vivid ways to celebrate the special days of your life right now. What fragrance signals birthdays to you? Is it the sweetness of vanilla or chocolate in a cake? Or is it something sophisticated, like night-blooming jasmine? What aroma indicates successful transitions, like a new job or a graduation? Would it be the burst of grapefruit or the explosion of a tingling orange?

Fragrances provide us with some of the most subtle and yet powerful ways for bringing back a sense of the past and giving us a deep appreciation of the present. In the chapters that follow, you will discover dozens of ways to use incense for creating enjoyable moods in your home, enhancing common activities, and setting the scene for meaningful, reflective moments, both alone and shared with others.

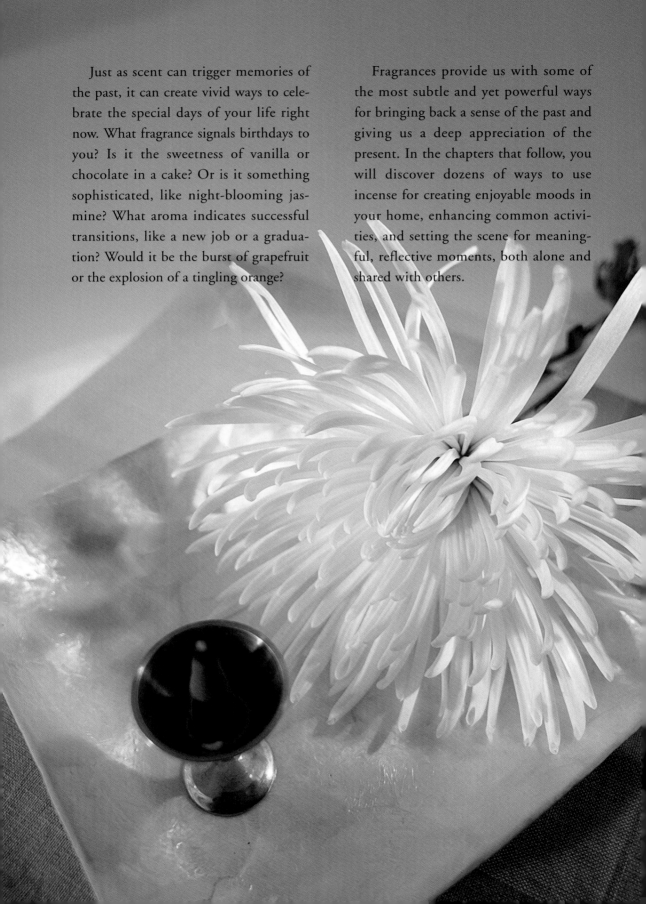

the mystery of Scent

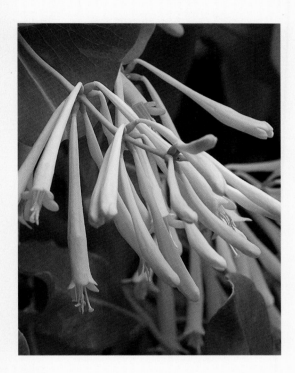

One fun way to develop scent awareness is to play a simple scent identification game. The Japanese have created countless charming games with the use of scent for their incense ceremonies.

This version of "guessing scents" is patterned after an old-fashioned treasure hunt. The objective of the game is to correctly name all the scents, and find them stashed in places in your house or in your garden.

Limiting the game to four scents (the nose can get overwhelmed by more), choose aromas that are not at all alike. For example, choose a citrus, a floral, a plant or tree, and something just for fun: tea, spices, chocolate, pineapple, or, to be funny, musty old shoes.

Write down a riddle or description of each. For example:

CLUE: "I am round and yellow and when I'm in Texas, I blush."

ANSWER: Pink grapefruit

CLUE: "I'm in the valley, small and white and many women take my name."

ANSWER: Lily of the valley

CLUE: "I am dusty and earthy, and have been the perfect gift for centuries."

ANSWER: Frankincense or myrrh

CLUES: "Christmas . . . a wood for shelves and cabinets . . . shaped like a cone."

ANSWER: Pine

Each player must first figure out the answers to these clues, then search through the home or garden for their representations. Rather than leave lit incense everywhere, leave something indicative of the scent: whole grapefruits, packages of myrrh cone incense, wreaths of pine, and stems of lily of the valley. The first person to collect them all wins!

Another way to play is to pass around fragrance sticks and have players close their eyes and try to guess the scent. If a player is stumped, more and more clues can be given until he or she comes up with the right answer.

Afterwards, everyone can come together to enjoy a convivial supper, where they can reveal where and how they figured out the clues and ferreted out the treasures. It's a little silly, a lot of fun, and a "scent-sational" way to kick off a party.

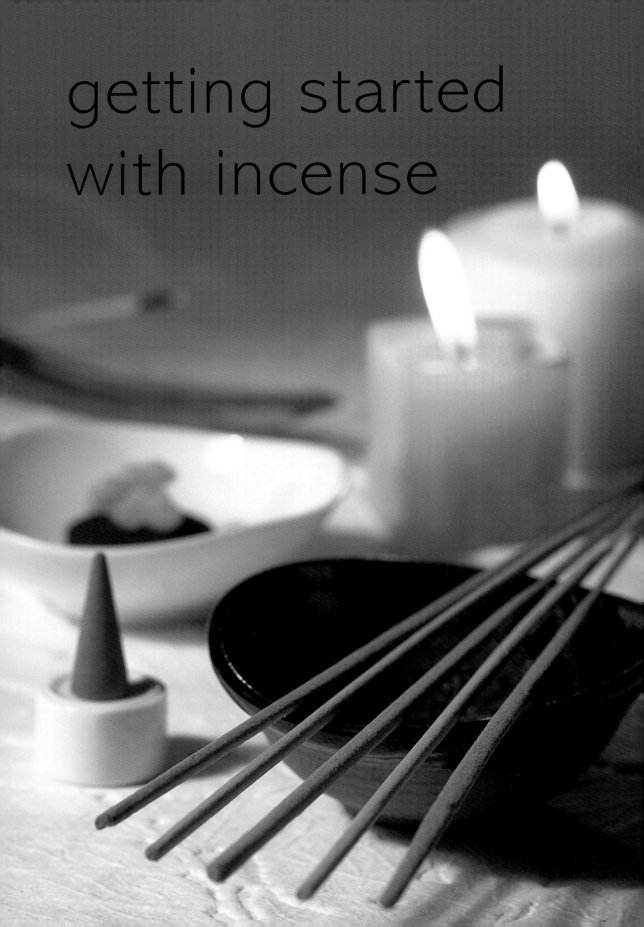

getting started
with incense

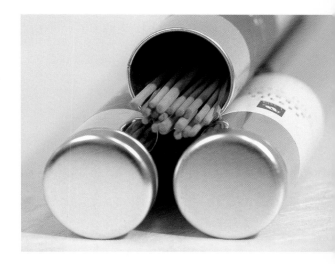

W alk into any store that carries a good supply of incense and what will strike you immediately — or right after the complex, intriguing scent all around you does — is the almost bewildering assortment of incense sticks, cones, powders, and accessories in all manner of shapes, colors, and sizes.

It can be a little intimidating, especially if you're not quite sure of the proper name and purpose for everything you see. That's why I've included here an incense primer, an introduction to the many varieties of incense and accessories available today.

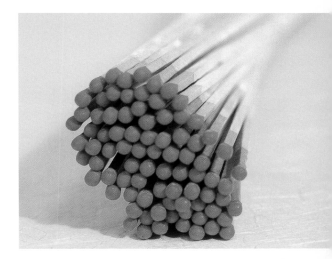

As you become more familiar with incense, you'll discover which varieties have the scents most pleasing to you, which forms of incense are the most convenient for you to use, and which have the most positive effects on your mood and spirit. Rather than feeling intimidated, you'll soon see how the world of incense is a place you can explore nearly endlessly, while still finding those small corners with just the right incense and accessory for any situation or need.

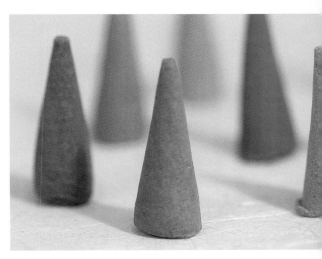

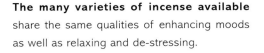

The many varieties of incense available share the same qualities of enhancing moods as well as relaxing and de-stressing.

Heavenly Fire

The term "joss stick" originated with the Chinese, who burned their fragrant paste sticks in a joss house or Chinese temple. The sticks are still commonly lit in front of a Chinese god or icon on home or temple altars as a way to "link heaven and earth." The Chinese believed fire itself was an act of cleansing, deflecting evil while its smoke attracted good spirits.

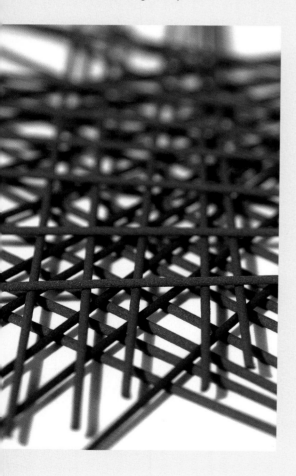

Varieties of Incense

Two types of incense are commonly available: combustible and noncombustible. The combustible type usually contains potassium nitrate (saltpeter) to aid in burning, while noncombustible incense does not.

Combustible incense can be burned in the form of cones, sticks, coils, or loose powder; noncombustible incense must be burned on glowing charcoal blocks or directly on a fire in order to release its fragrance.

Sticks

Also known as wands or fragrance sticks, this common form of incense is usually made of thin bamboo skewers coated with powdered kneaded incense. Sticks are available in all sizes and thicknesses and are perhaps the easiest incense to use. Many come with a little round or square piece of tile with a hole in the middle. Simply stand an incense stick in the hole, light the stick, lightly blow out the flame, and allow the smoke to scent the room.

An exception is joss sticks, which have no skewer at their center and are made of pure incense paste. They are delicate and generally purer in fragrance. Joss sticks are inexpensive, burn easily, and tend to scatter their fragrant ashes.

Coils

Coils are made the same way as joss sticks but are molded into spirals. They burn slowly and fragrantly and require ash catchers. Coils can be as small as two inches, or as large as two feet wide and one inch thick for burning in temples. Both Chinese and Japanese coil incenses are remarkably delicate and relaxing.

Cones

Cones are one of the most popular forms of incense in the world because they burn cleanly, require little in the way of accessories, and do not spill ashes everywhere. They are made by pressing powdered kneaded incense into cone-shaped molds. Pinion and cedar are popular ingredients for American-made cones; exquisite floral and light perfumes are common Japanese cone scents.

Noncombustibles

Noncombustible incense is usually smoldered over a small charcoal block placed in a censer or other fireproof container. Charcoal blocks are usually rectangular or round in shape and have potassium nitrate added to help them ignite; they should be kept away from moisture. Once the charcoal begins to glow, a half teaspoon or so of the incense is placed on the block. Types of

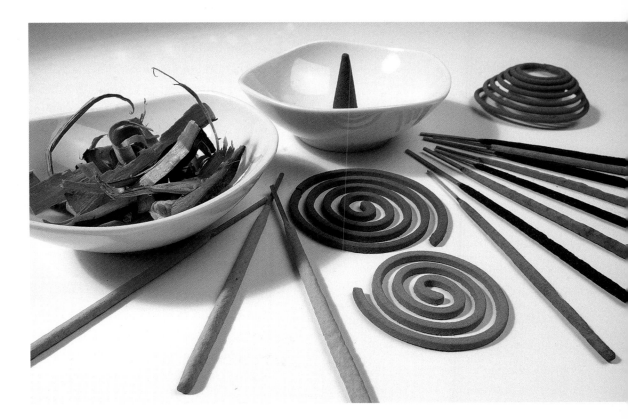

Incense Safety

Safety is of paramount importance when using incense in any form. Before lighting incense, make sure that there are no flammable items nearby.

* Avoid lighting incense in drafty areas. A breeze can carry sparks to flammable items.

* Be sure to extinguish matches completely in water. Never leave burning incense unattended, even for a second.

* When incense has burned completely, discard ashes in dirt, salt or sand, or saturate with water. Do NOT discard ashes in wastebaskets, as their heat may start a fire.

* Never leave burning charcoal unattended. After it burns out completely, pick it up with metal tongs or tweezers (not a potholder) and saturate it with water.

* ALWAYS keep all packaged and burning incense away from pets or children.

* Scent can be absorbed through the skin and into the blood. Please consult your physician before using incense or incense oils if you are pregnant or nursing a baby, have high blood pressure or any condition involving seizures, or have had a stroke.

noncombustible incense include longer-burning resins and gums such as frankincense and myrrh, or more fleeting varieties such as herbs, woods, or leaves.

In their incense ceremonies, the Japanese often light tiny pieces of fragrant wood known as *jin-koh,* which range from the size of a kernel of rice to about one inch across.

Incense Oils

Specially formulated essential oils are used to scent fragrance sticks or are added to lamp rings or to potpourri to scent a room. These are an excellent choice for those sensitive to smoke. Incense oils should not be handled with bare hands, as their intensity can irritate the skin.

Some essential oils are hazardous and should NOT be used in incense or aromatherapy applications. They are rue, brown and yellow camphor, bitter almond (synthesized as nitrobenzene), wormwood, sassafras, thuja, mugwort, pennyroyal, cinnamon leaf, and cassia. Rosemary, fennel, and hyssop oils can induce seizures in sensitive people.

Powders

For fun and charm, many incense manufacturers now shape incense powders into fanciful hearts, circles, flowers, animals, and many other forms. They're brilliantly colored, too, and both forms and powders are commercially available, if you would like to make your own.

if Smoke gets in your Eyes

There is no such thing as 100-percent smoke-free incense. Sloppy manufacture and synthetic or poor-quality ingredients will result in heavy, eye-watering smoke. But with careful production, exceptional ingredients, and care in handling, the result can be incense with very modest amounts of smoke.

Although some poorer countries make incense that looks rather rough, appearance is not much of a barometer for smokiness. Read the list of ingredients to be sure that the components are top-quality, and the incense is made from pure, raw elements. If smokiness bothers you, noncombustible incenses like scented woods or kneaded incense are better choices.

Ironically, incense of pure ingredients may be beneficial to people with asthma. However, anyone with a lung disease or a breathing disorder should consult a health professional prior to using incense. Although smoke from incense can be considered an indoor pollutant, the amount is so minimal that using incense is generally no more toxic than lighting candles. ✳

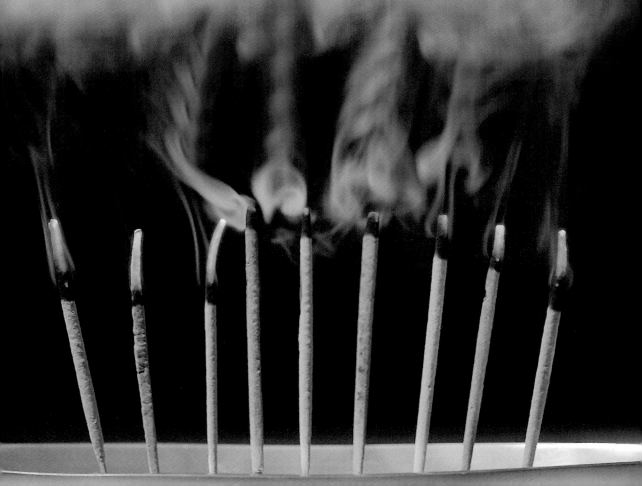

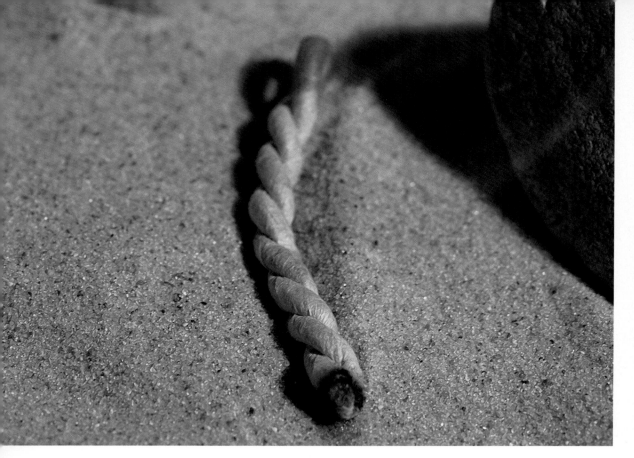

Ropes embellished with incense paste are lit by Tibetan monks as powerful carriers of prayers to the heavens.

Smudge Bundles

Used by many Native American tribes, bundles are dried herbs or grasses tied together with string or rope. One end is lit, then the fire is extinguished and the bundle is allowed to smoke over an ash catcher, usually an abalone shell or heatproof ceramic container.

The smudging is a result of rubbing the ashes on a surface or on the body. Sweetgrass or sage, the most common bundle ingredients, are excellent for purification of a home or the body. Some bundles contain lavender, or cedar or pinion chips.

Ropes

Himalayan rope incense is usually thick four-inch-long pieces of rope twisted together into a bundle. The rope bundle is coated with an incense mixture made of crushed herbs and powdered sandalwood, and the wonderful aroma when it is burned is very relaxing.

Most commonly found in Tibet, rope incense is made by Buddhist monks who believe that when it is burned, the smoke from ropes invites the deities to bring to all life happiness and peace.

Chipped Mixtures

Used at Buddhist altars, chipped mixtures include from five to ten ingredients: for example, a mixture of sandalwood,

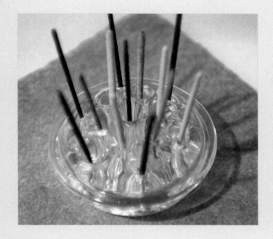

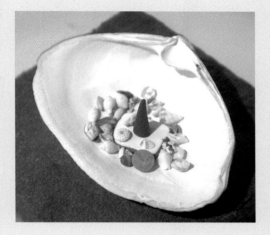

Flower or plant frogs are not images of Kermit, but the stands in which professional florists place stems for graceful displays. Frogs come in sizes from one to six inches in diameter, and either in glass with holes or with metal "grass."

Place the frog on a fireproof trivet, stick several incense sticks into it, and light as usual. The glass need not be heatproof, but ashes may fall onto the trivet, which should be fireproof.

The abalone shell is the traditional ash catcher for many Native American smudging and purification ceremonies, and large seashells are attractive natural accessories for your incense burning. For safety, place some sand, salt, or white ash in the body of the shell and place incense on top of that. Another safety measure is to put the shell on a fireproof trivet or plate.

Most salt and pepper shakers have holes just the right size for incense sticks (saltshakers tend to have larger holes than pepper shakers). Place the shaker on a fireproof plate or trivet, put one or more incense sticks into the holes, and light as usual. The ashes should fall onto the fireproof plate. This is a terrific idea for solitary shakers that have lost their mates.

Any heat-resistant, fireproof ceramic dishes such as tea-bag rests or soy sauce or salt dishes can be creative holders for cone incense. For extra drama, place the dish atop a box or stand and set the cone in the middle of the dish.

A long spoon rest makes a quirky holder for stick or wand incense. Lay the stick end on the "handle" of the spoon rest. Light the incense and its ashes will fall into the bowl of the rest. ✳

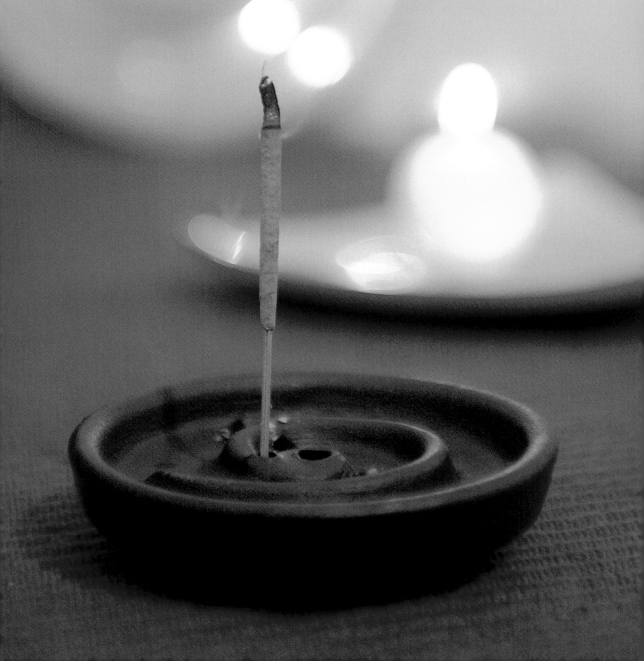

welcoming scents
for the home

If you've ever sold a house, you may have been advised to create the smells of home by boiling a pot of cinnamon on the stove or heating up bread in the oven to capture the interest of prospective buyers.

You don't have to be selling your house to have a reason for filling it with enticing aromas. Try burning a stick of a fragrance from the kitchen such as vanilla or chocolate, cinnamon, or clove to create the welcoming smell of home. Or opt for a fun, refreshing scent like watermelon, strawberry, or another fruity fragrance.

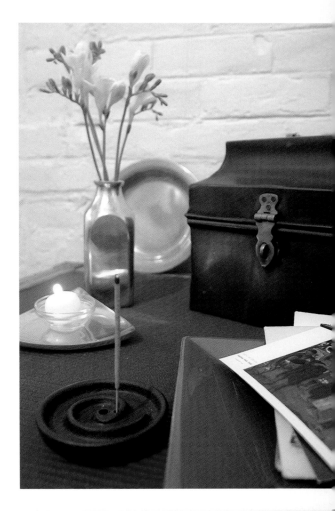

Why of seknesse deyeth man

While sawge in gardeyn

He may hav.

— *John Lelamoure, 1373*

modern variation:

how can a man die while he has Sage in his garden?

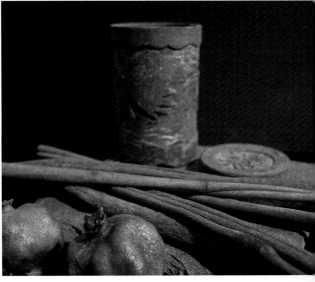

A fragrant stick of incense on an entry table (above right), perhaps an enticing scent such as cinnamon (right), will make guests feel immediately at home.

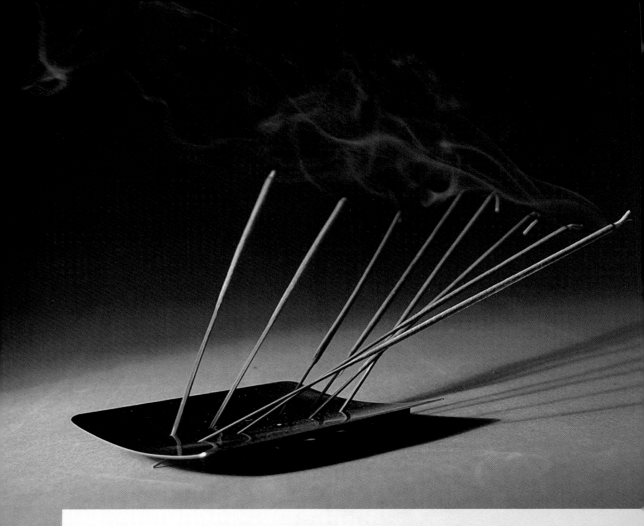

Blessing a New Home

One meaningful way to mark the transition when you move into a new house is to burn incense as part of a simple housewarming ceremony witnessed by family and friends. This symbolic act invites the blessings of spirit to enter and reside in your home. You might think of it as clearing away the old lethargy and complacency that may have occupied the house and making way for new, fresh energy and life.

A home blessing doesn't have to be reserved for a move. It can be useful at other times of change as well, whether it's a new season, a child's moving out to attend college or live on her own, or a redirecting of your life's purpose. Purifying a home with incense is an especially lovely gesture to usher in the Sabbath day, a new year, an anniversary, or whatever other occasions are significant to you.

You may have ideas for developing a simple ceremony that reflects your cultural, religious, or spiritual beliefs. Or you can adapt a traditional housewarming custom from another culture to create a new tradition of your own.

Sweetgrass and sage are the traditional Native American scents associated with purification. The soft, sweet fragrance of sweetgrass is reminiscent of the scent of vanilla. Sweetgrass grows tall and is often braided into bundles, called smudge sticks, that produce an intense aroma when lit. Sage is also available in ready-made bundles; these should be flexible and highly aromatic to indicate freshness.

To use as incense, light one end of the bundle, then blow out the flame. As the bundle continues to smoke, hold an abalone shell or clay bowl underneath to catch the ashes. Go to each room of your new home, making sure to scent each of its four corners to reflect the four directions: east, west, north, and south. Ask for blessings and peace for all who will live here and for those who enter as loving visitors.

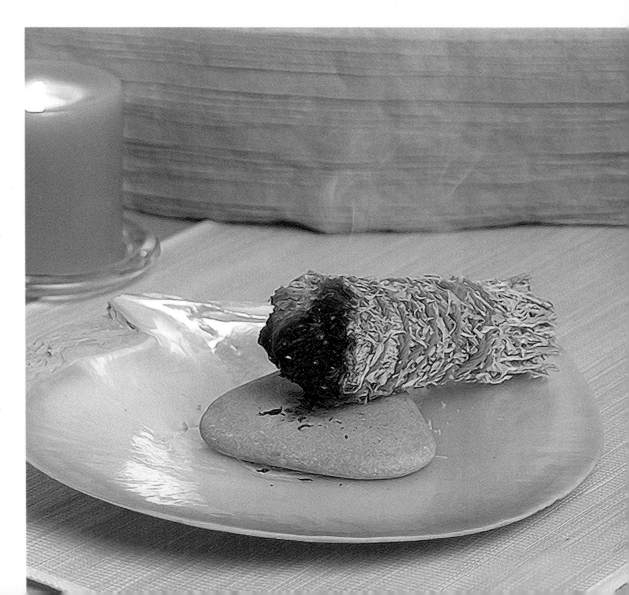

Fragrant Greetings

For centuries, sage has provided a traditional scent for ceremonies of purification and for blessing a new home. Start your own tradition by placing a combination of crushed dried sage leaves and sage incense underneath your doormat. As your family and visitors cross the threshold, the fresh, cleansing scent of sage will enter the house with them.

Creating a Home Altar

An altar serves as a focal point for spirituality in your home, whether it's a place to connect with nature, with those people or activities you love, or with your religious beliefs. It can take many forms. You may not realize it, but you probably already have some type of altar in your home: photos of loved ones displayed on a mantel or dresser, special shells and rocks collected on family vacations arranged on a windowsill, or even your refrigerator door covered with artwork children made years ago.

To create or expand your home altar, reflect on what inspires your spiritual life. It might be a religious icon or object,

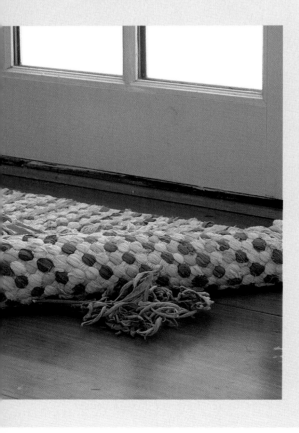

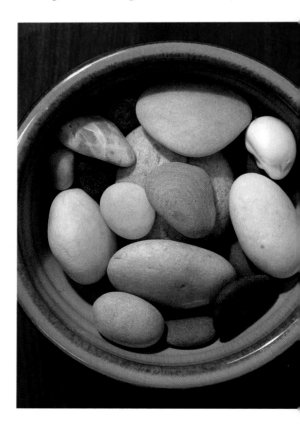

such as a saint, a prayer book, a cross, Sabbath candles, or a figure of a Buddha. Or your altar may be totally sectarian, featuring photos of spouses, parents, children, or even a drawing or photo of your home itself. It may change and evolve to reflect your needs at a particular time.

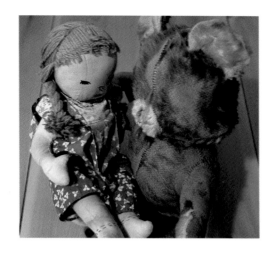

If your raggedy teddy bear still centers you, let him sit on your altar when you need him. An altar doesn't have to be totally serious; if that plastic windup toy reminds you of your best friend, on the altar it goes. Does your child's favorite dolly or model airplane sing to you? Add it. Is your home undergoing the chaos of remodeling? Put an artifact, a magazine clipping, or even the contractor's agreement on the altar and say prayers for timely and beautiful completion.

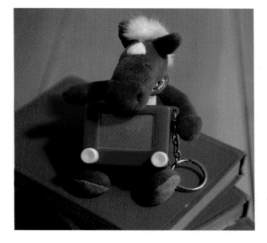

Anything that you treasure belongs on your home altar, from a favorite childhood toy to stones and shells from a memorable trip.

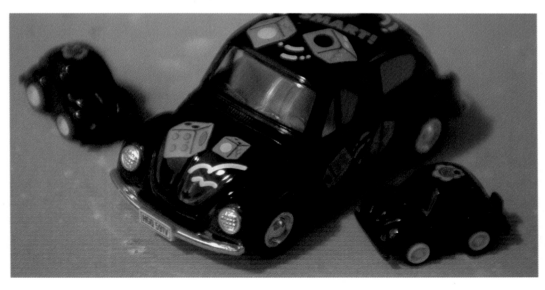

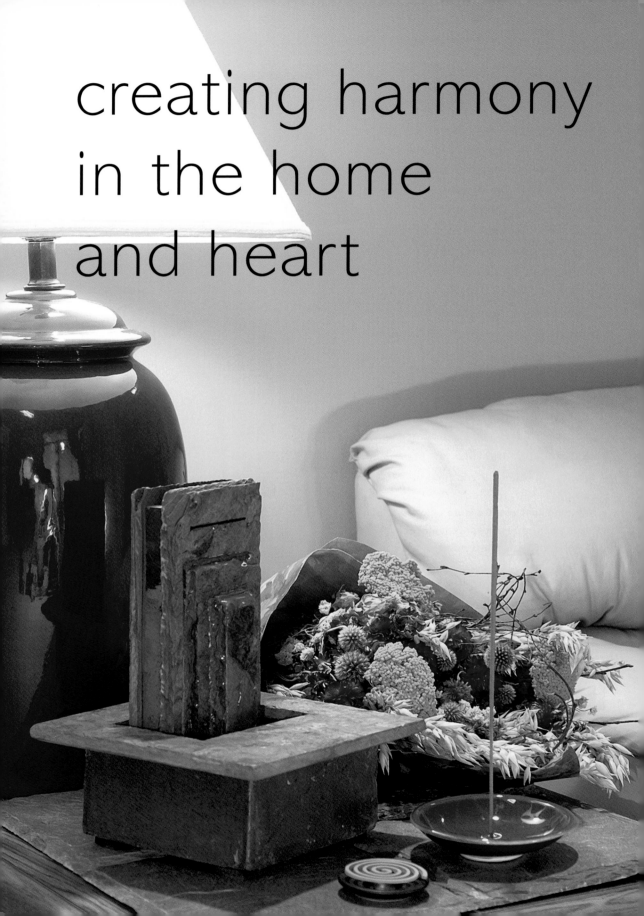

creating harmony
in the home
and heart

Just as incense clears the stagnant air in a home or repels illness or bad vibrations, it can clear the air following a disagreement or an argument and help bring forth healing thoughts and prayers.

Sandalwood incense has been used for more than 4,000 years to calm the mind, enhance mental clarity, and open the gateway to the spiritual (or, as it is known in ancient Eastern philosophy, the Third Eye, or brow chakra). Sandalwood is believed to help relieve insomnia, abate depression, and ease anxiety and grief. Its sweet, woodsy scent is effective in calming even the most agitated feelings.

Sandalwood may be the most common element in the serene incense sticks of Japan and in the subtle to bold incense of India. It is likely the most predominant incense scent in the world.

Other scents for comfort and healing are those in the traditional Tibetan healing sticks, such as frankincense, myrrh, cedar, pine, and pinion.

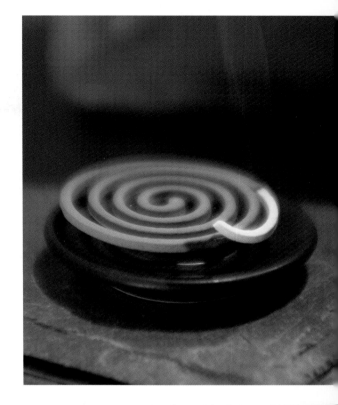

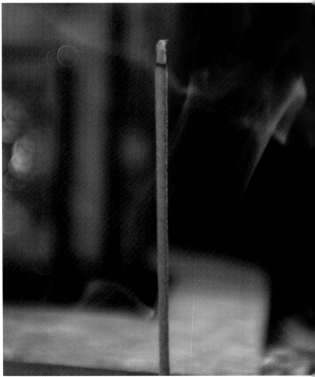

In a dark time,
the eye begins to see.
Theodore Roethke
(U.S. poet, 1908–1963)

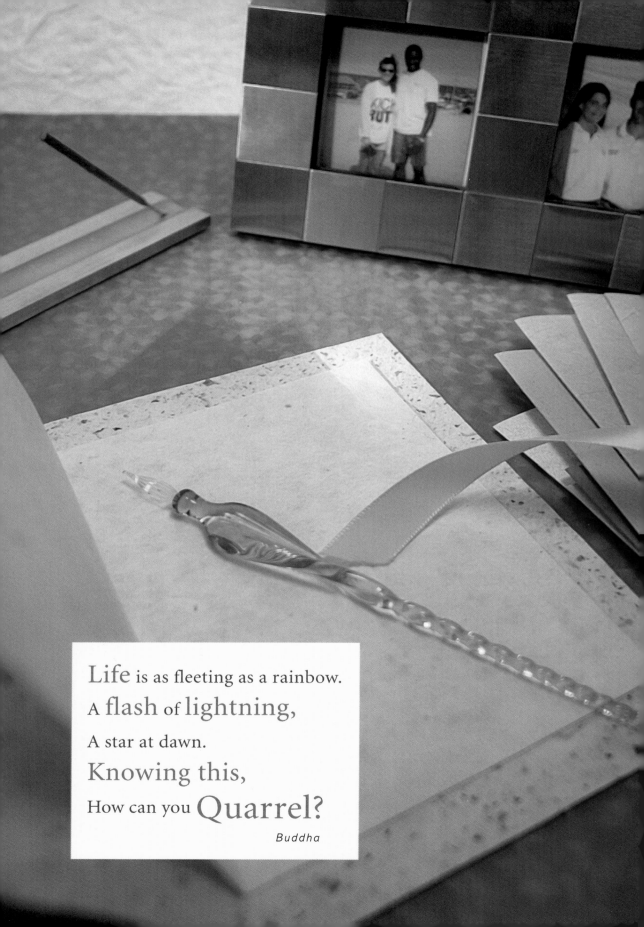

Life is as fleeting as a rainbow.
A flash of lightning,
A star at dawn.
Knowing this,
How can you Quarrel?

Buddha

Opening to Healing

Healing a rift with someone close to you often requires an initial period of reflection on what has disturbed the relationship and what will bring reconciliation. How can we open our hearts? What will ease our minds and soothe our bodies? Lighting incense, particularly one with a fragrance connected with comfort, such as sandalwood, can help create a soothing atmosphere for such reflection. Choose a quiet place, perhaps where the disagreement took place. Or you might sit in front of your home altar with symbols before you of the relationship that needs healing. These symbols can be letters, photos, pages from your journal, anything that speaks of the person or persons involved.

Light the incense. Breathe in its therapeutic scent. Lift up your shoulders and roll them three times forward and three times backward until they are fully relaxed. Allow the incense to burn out completely.

Sometimes we don't know why or how division has pushed us away from the people or places we care about. Separation sometimes just happens. Other times we remember harsh words, misunderstandings, and exclusions from the fold. It all hurts, but the pain does not have to last forever.

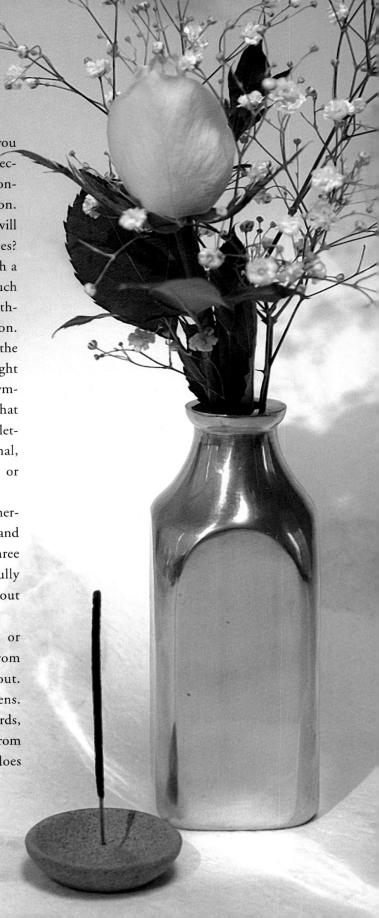

Beginning Anew

A phone call, a letter, even an e-mail, can be the beginning of erasing the line of separation. As long as the goal is pure, coming together again can happen.

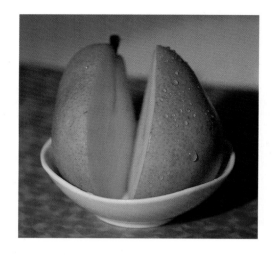

Choose an incense fragrance that is completely new to you. Try one that is pleasant and light to reflect your cleansing, perhaps a citrus scent, which is associated with fresh energy. You might enjoy one of the delightful fragrance sticks imbued with a fruit aroma such as mango, strawberry, melon, berry, or pear. By opening yourself up to something as simple as a different fragrance, you begin the path to other changes. In your own way, ask for the strength and clarity to bring about change in your life and your relationships.

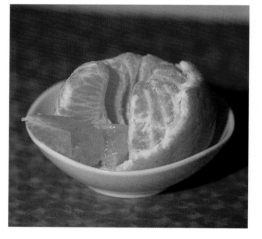

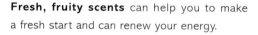

Fresh, fruity scents can help you to make a fresh start and can renew your energy.

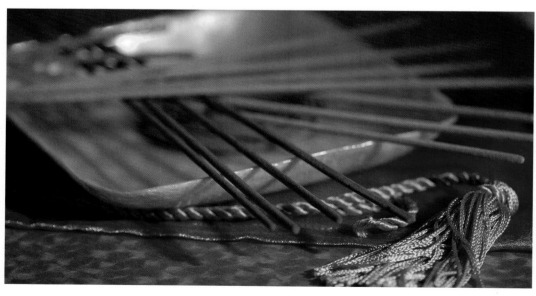

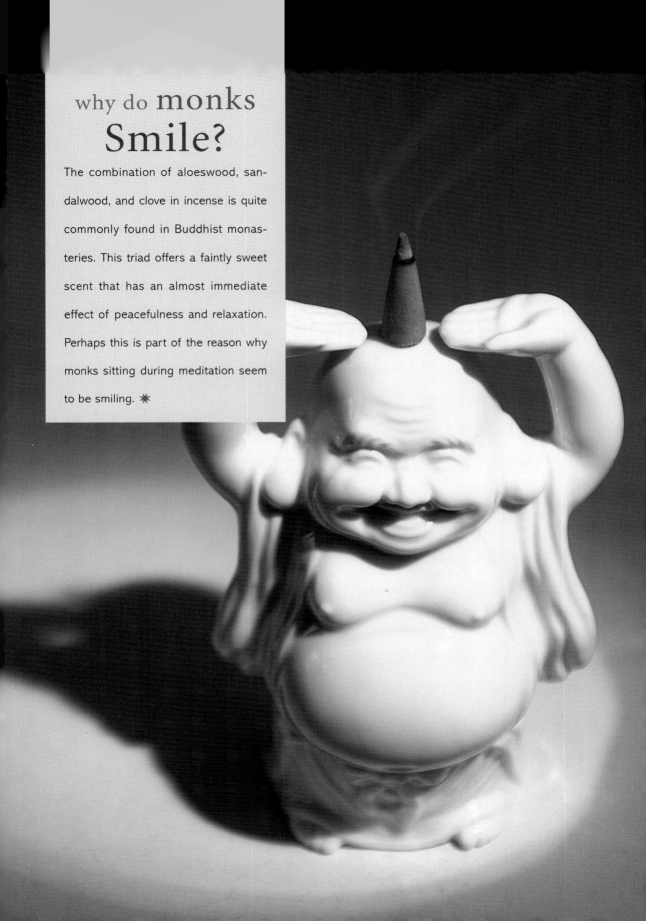

why do monks
Smile?

The combination of aloeswood, sandalwood, and clove in incense is quite commonly found in Buddhist monasteries. This triad offers a faintly sweet scent that has an almost immediate effect of peacefulness and relaxation. Perhaps this is part of the reason why monks sitting during meditation seem to be smiling. ✳

Fragrances for Renewed Friendship

A reunion to mend a friendship or renew a lapsed relationship is enhanced by incense. Ask your friend to help you create a friendship altar from items each of you brings that delight, charm, or recall pleasurable times spent together: photos, toys, favorite gifts, food, or drink.

Choose incense that reflects favorite scents like the sharpness of cinnamon or clove or the sweetness of vanilla or chocolate. Who can resist the aroma of hot chocolate or the tang of apples with cinnamon? These familiar smells will bring back pleasant memories to help the process of reunion and reconnection.

As you light the incense, take turns explaining the significance of the gifts you brought to the friendship altar and your hopes for the future. Allow the incense to embrace both of you, and to take you to a place of forgiveness, reconciliation, and new beginning.

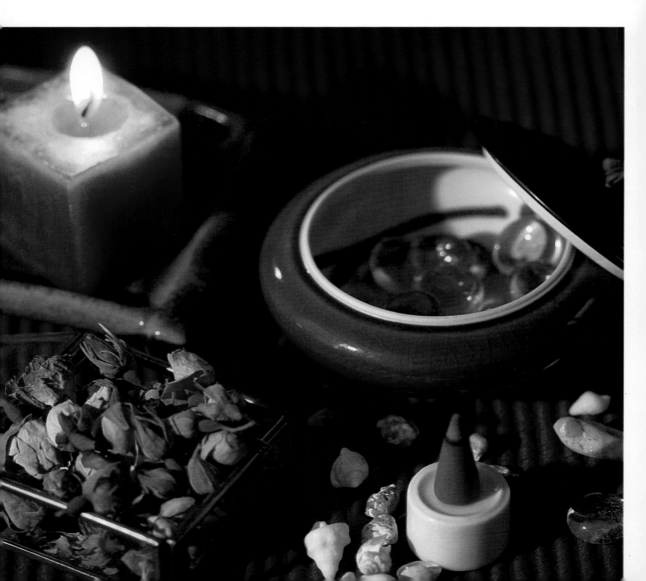

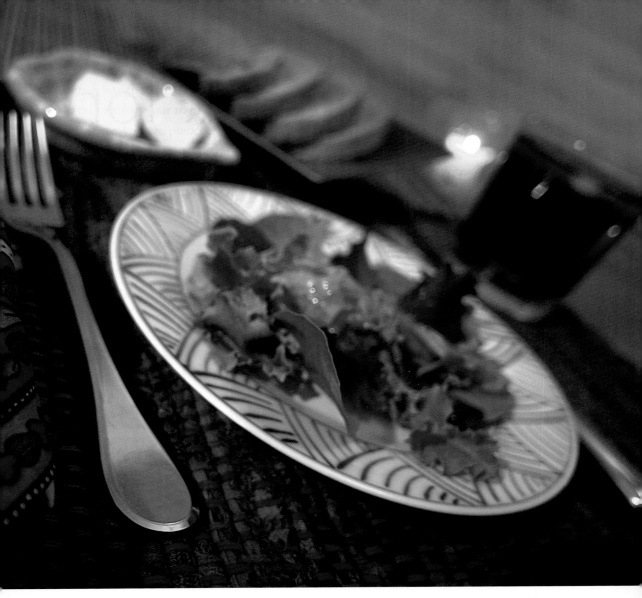

Enjoying a delicious, fragrant meal together can be the first step in a renewed relationship.

It requires a strong desire to place friendship above ego to say, "I was wrong." It takes a mature soul to accept a changed heart without blame. Reaching this level of compassion for the weakness, the humanity in all of us brings enormous benefits: a release from the grief of division and the second chance we all desire.

When the words have ceased and the incense has burned away, close your eyes and feel the sense of peace give way to newfound energy.

Now is the time to make plans for the future! Celebrate in the way of the ancients: Break bread, toast each other, revel in the exquisite pleasure of a growing appreciation and love for each other.

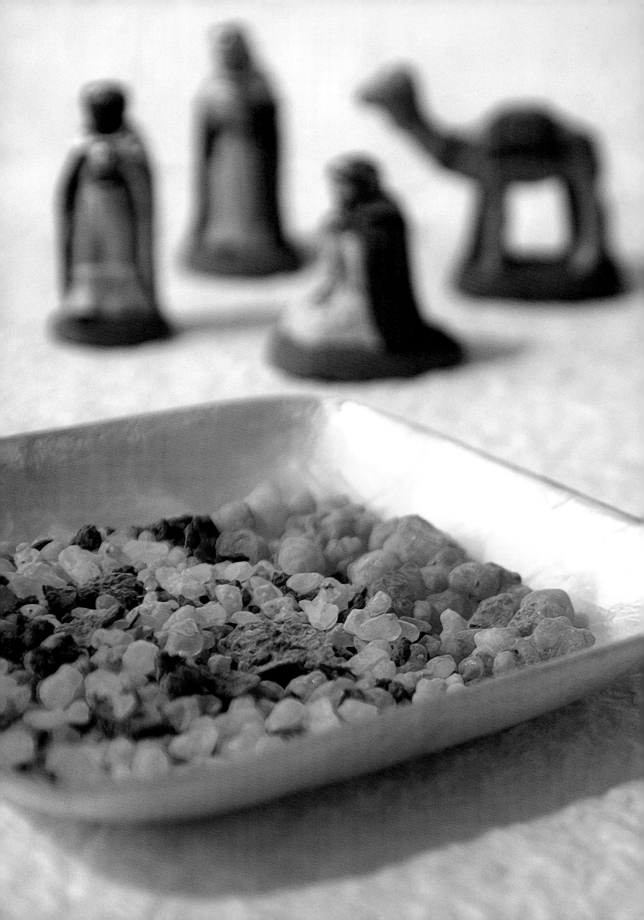

Fragrances for Quiet Reflection

Frankincense is the original fragrance for meditation, the fragrance of peace. Its sweet, woodsy smokiness is said to produce a substance that expands the subconscious without any negative after-effects, a suitable stimulant for the energy center that is known as the crown, or seventh, chakra, which is associated with enlightenment.

Frankincense is best known as one of the gifts (along with myrrh and gold) brought by the three Magi in honor of the birth of Christ. In some cultures, frankincense is the very word used for incense in general. Its earthy, woodsy scent effectively transports even the most distressed person into a sense of calm, and its fragrance purifies, cleanses, and prepares you to enter a new day.

Its sister surely is myrrh, which also has a dusty, woodsy scent and a calming effect. Research has been done recently on the possible therapeutic benefits of myrrh in fighting some debilitating diseases.

According to some scholars, balsam and ambergris were also among the gifts of the Magi. These are both classic elements in perfume, providing muskiness and heaviness to incense fragrances that need more body and fullness.

frankincense along the Incense road

During the 10th century, the kingdom of Sheba grew both myrrh and frankincense to such an extent that its entire economy relied upon these precious resins. A caravan trail, known as the Incense Road, developed as the route from which Sheba merchants carried these resins to Egypt, perhaps the most avid consumer of oils, perfumes, and incense the world has ever known.

When it was obvious how expensive these gum resins were, the caravans of frankincense-laden camels were frequently hijacked by enterprising thieves. Many historians now believe the real reason the Queen of Sheba sought out King Solomon was to obtain his protection of her Incense Road and the valuable cargo that traversed it. ✳

give yourself a simple
brain-balancing Massage

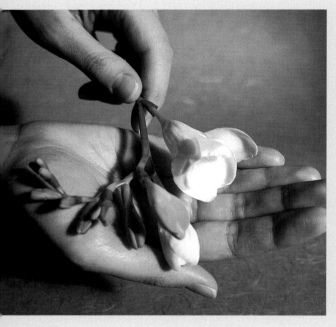

This simple head massage affects the seventh, or crown, chakra, which affects the vital life force of the body, the immune system. It is believed to increase the efficacy of the pineal gland, located on top of your head.

The massage takes only a few minutes, and it will almost immediately help bring nourishing blood to the brain and naturally stimulate it. This simple physical act opens the gate to reflection and can be done anywhere, anytime. Tapping into our energy flows can be mental or physical. This gentle exercise starts energy flowing immediately.

1 **Light frankincense** in a burner, then gently blow out the flame. Wave a feather or your hand over the burning edge of the incense to fan it slightly and keep it burning. Inhale this ephemeral, delicately woodsy smoke of the ages; realize that what you smell is the same scent that fascinated the ancient Egyptians, Greeks, and Romans. This is the same scent inhaled by Abraham, Isaac, and Jacob, and a part of the triumvirate of gifts from the Magi on that first Christmas.

2 As this timeless aroma permeates the room, allow yourself to submit to its power. **Be calmed**, be transported to a level of genuine relaxation, be at peace in silence.

3 **Curve your fingers** inward toward you and, beginning in the middle of your forehead, tap gently. Move the fingers to the side of your head, as if you were opening up your brain. Tap gently.

4 Next, start at the top of your head and **move your fingers down to the temples.** Tap gently.

5 Make the same gesture from the top of your head to the bottom of the back of your skull. **Tap one more time.**

You can do this exercise using the five steps here, or perform a simpler version without tapping. Move your fingers to the temples and rest for a few moments. By just allowing the energy points on the tips of your fingers to rest on your skin, you can transmit warmth and energy to your skin and help yourself relax. Next, move your fingers from the top of your head down the back of your head to the top of your neck. Rest your fingers at your nape. Feel the warmth emanating from your fingertips, and notice how it relaxes you.

With your eyes closed, imagine yourself opening up to the world and all its possibilities. Rest quietly for a few more moments to still your mind and allow reflection on the mystery of life and your connection to it.

Now open your eyes. Feel how refreshed and energized you have become. Sit quietly for another few minutes, allowing this wonderful new feeling to wash over you.

Extinguish the incense and continue with your day, more alert, more aware, ready for more wonder.

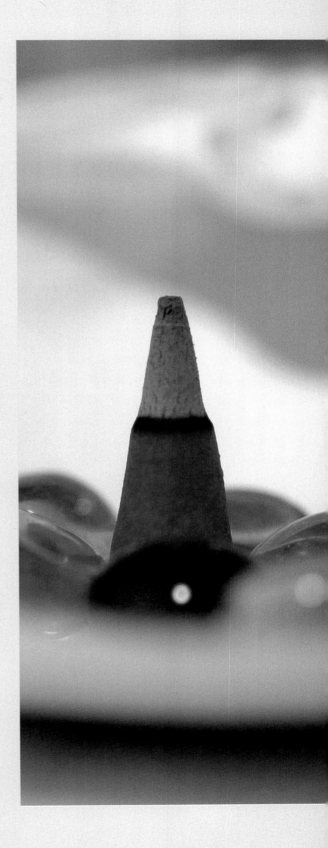

Sweet Dreams

Fragrances have long been considered the pathway to dreams. You can make a small dream pillow, about five inches by seven inches, and fill it with crushed dried violet leaves along with some crushed violet incense sticks or powder. Place it under your regular bed pillow or just inside the pillowcase. Whenever you move your head on the pillow, it will slightly crush the dried flowers and incense bits, releasing their subtle floral aroma, and help induce or sustain sleep. Lavender is an excellent sleep-inducing fragrance, too.

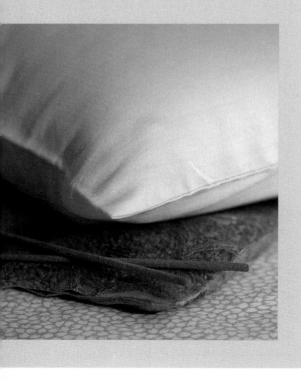

60,000 roses are needed to press out a mere 30 ml of essential oil. The Himalayan, Kashmir, and heirloom English roses are considered the sweetest and most delicate. Today, Bulgaria, France, Turkey, and Morocco grow the most roses for essential oil.

Although roses are the international favorite of lovers, jasmine, neroli (a citrus), lilies, and the Oriental lotus are frequently associated with the pleasures of the bedroom. An alternative is frankincense, whose mystic odor is believed to awaken sexual energy.

Seductive Scents for the Bed

Incense has a way of relaxing the body so that desire increases and love deepens. To set the mood in your bedroom, fold down the comforter to expose the sheets, and then strew soft petals from fresh roses upon the sheets. They will impart their exquisite fragrance as you lie upon them and will be silky smooth and sensuous against your skin. Next, light several candles at different heights nearby, pink and red if possible.

Play soft instrumental music that both you and your partner enjoy. Light a stick of rose incense. You might also set a diffuser lightbulb ring on a bedroom table lamp and add a few drops of rose oil before you turn it on. If you have a fireplace, consider tossing in a cone of incense to add a lovely touch of scent along with the warmth and flickering light of the flames in the hearth.

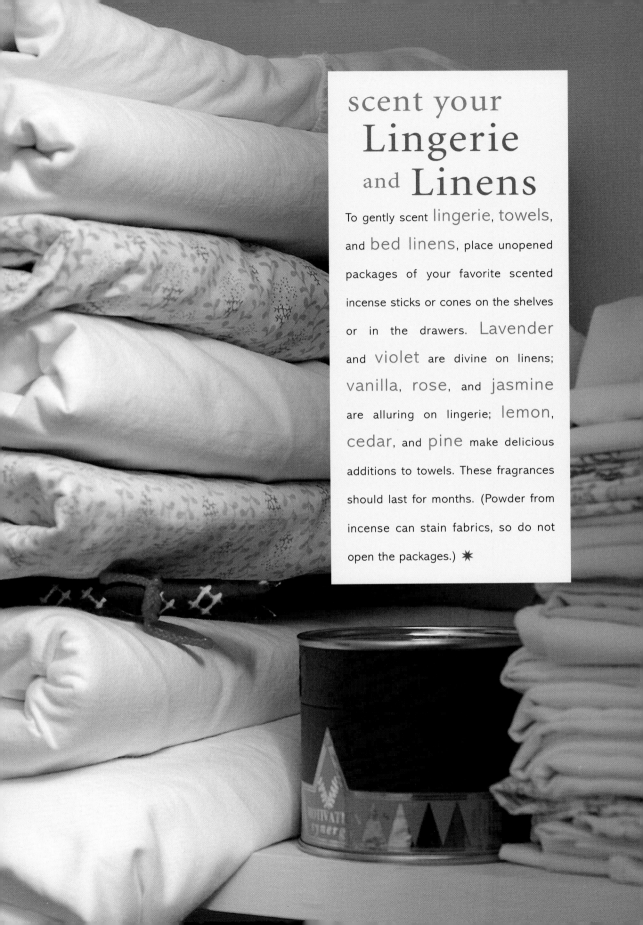

scent your Lingerie and Linens

To gently scent lingerie, towels, and bed linens, place unopened packages of your favorite scented incense sticks or cones on the shelves or in the drawers. Lavender and violet are divine on linens; vanilla, rose, and jasmine are alluring on lingerie; lemon, cedar, and pine make delicious additions to towels. These fragrances should last for months. (Powder from incense can stain fabrics, so do not open the packages.) ✳

a meditation for Lovers

Although meditation is generally a solitary method for stilling the mind, it can also be a powerful way to connect with another person. Find a comfortable seated position, either facing each other or sitting back-to-back. If you are comfortable with the cross-legged yoga sitting position, that is ideal, but you can also do this exercise sitting on a pillow on the floor, or sitting in a straight-backed chair.

In all meditation, concentration on breathing and on clearing the mind of intrusive thoughts is important to relax both the mind and the body.

1 **Begin by standing.** Light a stick of rose-infused incense. When the stick's fragrance begins to waft up, pick up the stick and walk around your partner three times. Then, passing the stick, ask your partner to walk around you three times.

2 **Place the incense** on a table and sit down again.

3 **Breathing through your nose,** inhale deeply, feeling the expansion of your lungs. Breathe out through your mouth, feeling the contraction of your abdomen as you expel the breath. Do this four times. If sitting back-to-back, be aware of your partner's breathing patterns; you may be able to duplicate the rhythm, but it is not necessary. Just being aware of your partner's presence is enough.

4 **See if you can sense** each other's energy points (called *chi* in Chinese and *ki* in Japanese). Feel your own energy centered within your body.

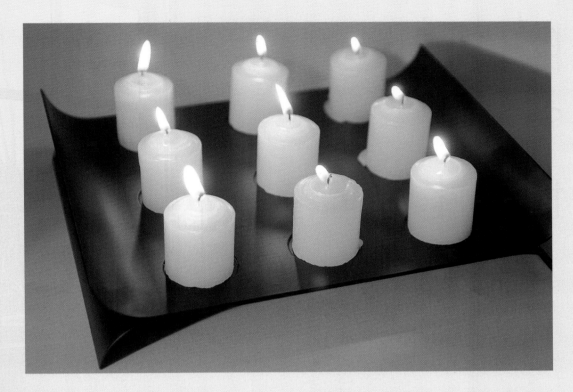

As you sit, try this simple visualization. Imagine a fire in your lower abdomen, feel the heat it radiates inside you increasing with every breath you take. Breathe in and out deeply. Think of the fire warming all of your body: first downward toward your hips, thighs, legs; then moving upward to your chest, arms, and head. Continue to breathe in and out in a relaxed manner. Repeat the steps, only this time, imagine the fire gradually cooling, until your body itself cools back to its usual temperature. This experience should leave you relaxed, comforted, and at peace.

The hand-in-hand peace gesture is another very effective way to diffuse tension between couples. The exercise can be done standing face-to-face with your partner or sitting on chairs face-to-face. Just be careful not to cross your legs, as it will divert your energy.

Close your eyes and, with your arms at your side, focus your energy and thoughts on the palms of your hands. Think of the most peaceful scene you can imagine: the stillness of a pond, the majesty of a mountaintop, the purity of snow, the glory of the sun or moon.

Imagine a warm wind of healing energy and send this directly to your palms until you feel a change, an increase in energy or heat in the curve of your palms. Slowly reach out for your partner's hands and repeat the exercise, this time sending energy, warmth, healing to him. Feel the connection of the energy between each other. Do this for as long as it feels comfortable. Your partner can then transmit his energy to you.

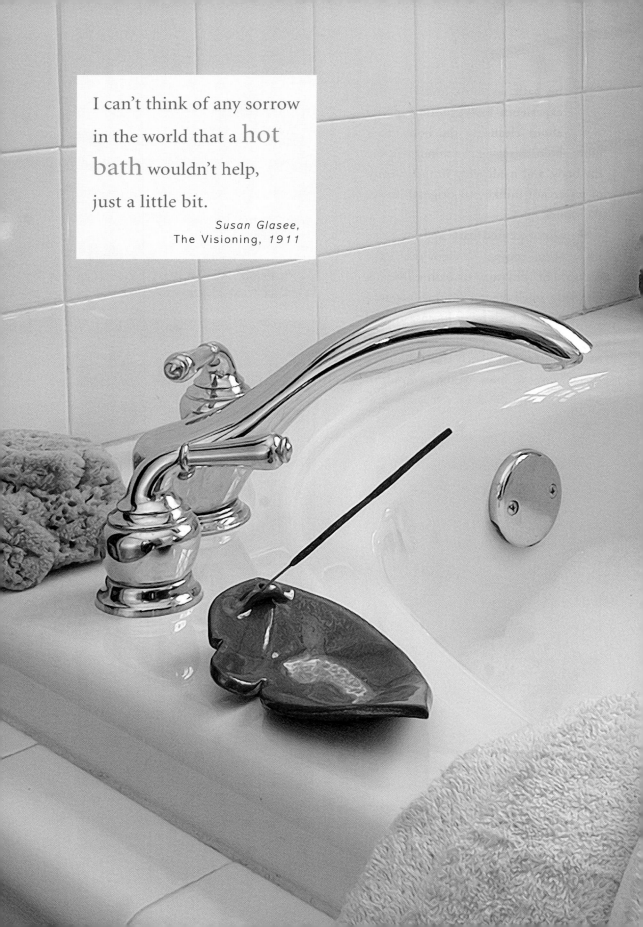

I can't think of any sorrow in the world that a **hot bath** wouldn't help, just a little bit.

Susan Glasee,
The Visioning, 1911

Fragrances to Cleanse and Relax

Lavender is the perfect scent for the bathroom, because it is very clean and refreshing. Even the word lavender is related to bathing, as it comes from the Latin word *lavare,* "to wash." Lavender has been used since the days of ancient Rome to scent baths and to sprinkle as lavender water *(eau de lavande)* on bed linens and toweling to induce relaxation and a restful sleep.

Sweet violets, Oriental jasmine, and rose absolute are equally relaxing. For the exotic or sensuous bath, consider ylang-ylang or gardenia; to refresh and awaken the body and spirit, try rosemary, lemon, or rosewood. Eucalyptus and pine are bracing scents perfect for a hot soak on a cold day. Sandalwood and frankincense are more contemplative, while nothing is sexier for many than vanilla and chocolate, perhaps the two most popular elements of scented products today.

It does not matter how simple or elegant your tub is. As long as the water is warm, the lights dim with only a candle or two burning, and the incense fragrance of your choice scenting the room gently, you can float away until you are thoroughly refreshed and relaxed.

Cleaning the bathtub before you bathe does much for enhancing the total experience. When you are through bathing, leave the tub cleaning for the next time, thus avoiding an abrupt halt to your floating experience.

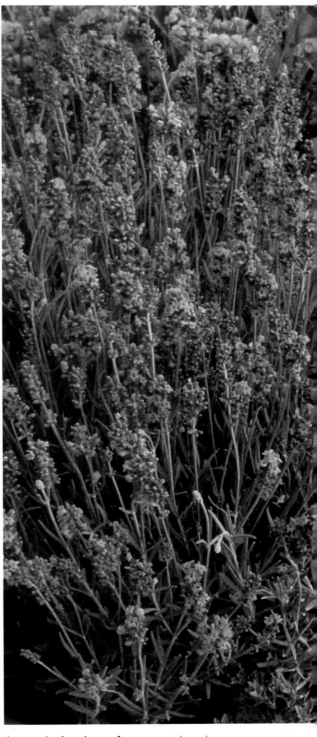

Lavender's clean fragrance has been a favorite in the bath and bedroom for centuries.

Room Refreshers

A simple, wonderful combination of function and form, incense matches are used exactly like ordinary matches: You strike them, and the flame ignites a small area of incense powder. The scent lasts just a short time, but long enough to whisk away any unpleasant odors. Discard them carefully in sand, or douse them with water.

Incense matches are better than breathing in the sulfur residue from regular matches, and better than aerosol room deodorants, which are usually almost all artificial ingredients. These matches are available at many of the places that sell incense, such as New Age and home fragrance departments in health food stores and accessories shops. They are available in frankincense, jasmine, fruity blends, and other classic incense fragrances.

An alternative to incense matches for quickly bringing a pleasant fragrance into your bathroom is to break off half- or one-inch pieces of incense coils or sticks and burn them in a small dish. The burning time is brief, and the fragrant effect is immediate. ✳

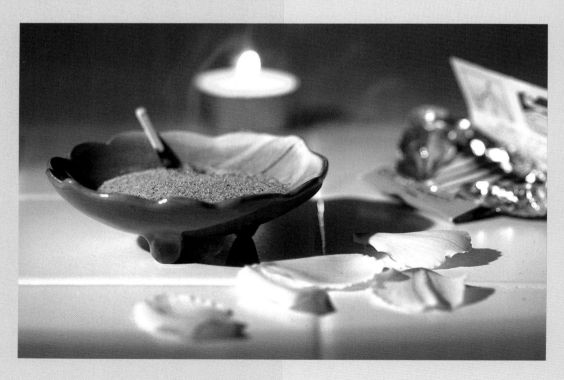

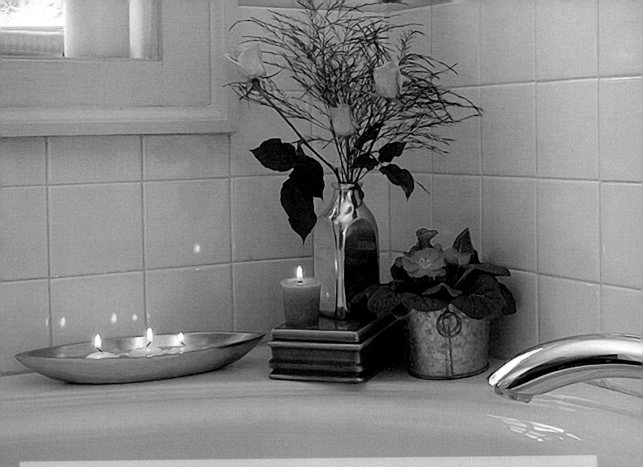

The Stress-Relief Bath

Set out freshly laundered towels. While the tub is filling up, light a few candles around the room, then light a lavender-imbued fragrance stick, making sure to place it in a safe area, away from curtains and towels. Unwrap your special soaps: luxurious shea butter or rich milk-based ones, or a milk-based bath powder to create unscented but voluminous bubbles to caress your skin while you soak.

As you disrobe, feel the steam and heat caress your body. Slowly and carefully, step into the bathtub, sit down, then lean back, making sure a rolled-up towel or inflatable pillow is cradling your neck in comfort.

Feel the warmth of the water covering each part of your body, from your toes to your ankles, calves, thighs, belly, chest, arms, and neck. Breathe in the lavender and relax your body.

If the warmth of the water is not relaxing enough on its own, practice this exercise: Beginning with your legs, tense your body while you inhale deeply, then relax. Move up to your thighs, buttocks, chest, and arms, tensing first, inhaling deeply, then exhaling as you release the tension. After this exercise, combined with the enveloping warmth of the tub water, you will be totally relaxed.

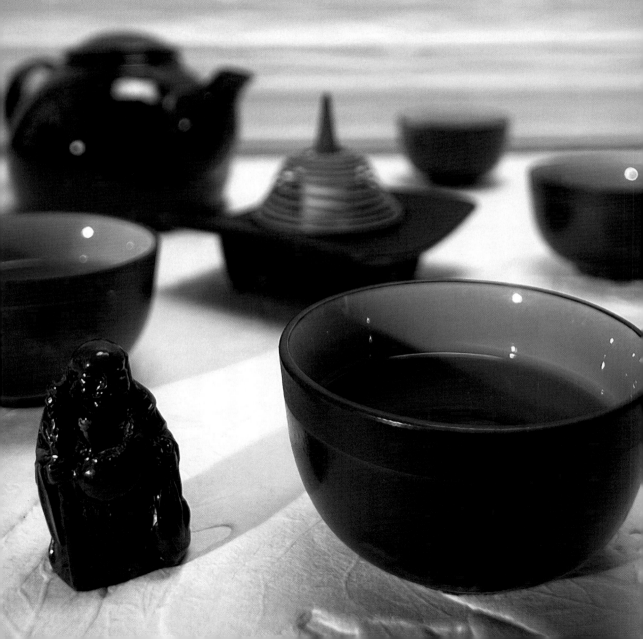

take a
zen vacation
with afternoon tea

Tea is perhaps the most soothing beverage when you want to take a break from life's daily routine. It is perfect for some time alone, sharing a relaxing moment with colleagues at work, connecting with friends, or just enjoying the company of family and other loved ones in the sanctity of your home. Its hot silky feel in the mouth, its fragrant bouquet, even the warmth of the cup in your hands, all contribute to the comfort and relaxation associated with a cup of tea.

The many practices surrounding the brewing and serving of tea throughout the world are as fascinating and as diverse as the types of tea available. Add the exquisite delicacy of a light lotus or jasmine incense to the satisfaction of drinking tea and you do, indeed, have the best of all worlds — a Zen vacation, if just for a moment.

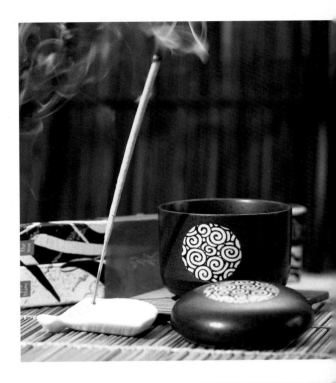

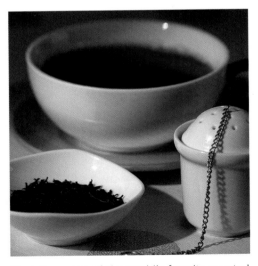

Earl Grey, one of the world's favorite scented teas, is a heady choice for incense.

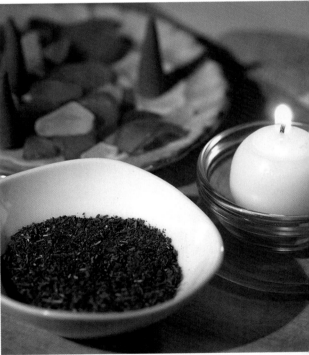

Green tea is now found in everything from cosmetics and bath products to incense.

Tea in Incense

Tea is as soothing as an ingredient in incense as it is in your teacup. Consider such varieties of tea-infused incense as jasmine, with its deeply floral note; Lapsang souchong, a smoky black tea; black teas with sweet fruits like pear, mango, passion fruit, or bergamot; the traditional flavor of Earl Grey; or unscented teas like black, oolong, or green.

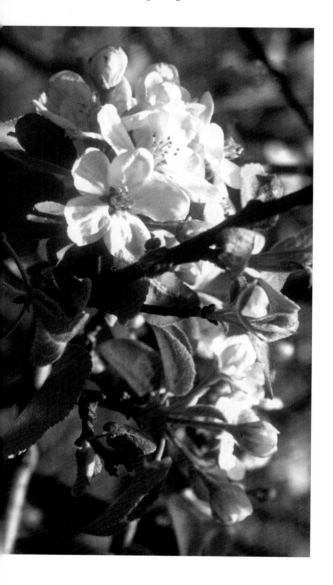

Should you be able to find it, neri-koh, the special kneaded, aged Japanese incense made with plum meat, is expressly meant for the tea ceremony and would be a unique and welcome addition to this Zenlike experience. Another choice is the aloeswood incense coils made in Japan; these offer a delicate, relaxing essence that will not overpower the aroma of your tea.

If you're hosting guests for tea, light a fragrance stick of your favorite incense in the foyer as a welcoming gesture before they arrive. This is a quiet, subtle way to set the mood, a subconscious signal for guests to relax and enjoy themselves. It is especially lovely to do this near your garden entrance when you have guests walking in and out of your home. Select an incense that will put your guests at ease, such as a tea-scented incense or the lighter, more delicate florals like lotus, fine rose, or lily.

Preparing a cozy cup of tea just for yourself? Light a stick of tea-scented incense as you put the water on to boil. Use the preparatory moments to inhale the sweet fragrance and enter fully into the contentment of the tea experience.

Exquisite jasmine (at left) adds an intoxicating, memorable scent to incense that makes for a perfect gesture of welcome.

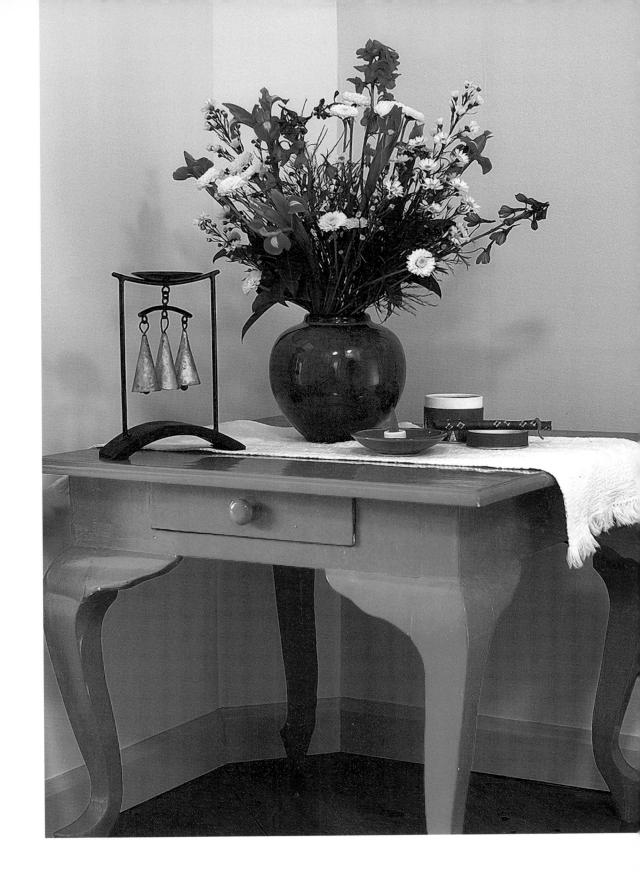

What's Your Tea Style?

The accoutrements for tea service contribute so much to creating the mood for your Zen vacation. Imagine having tea at Buckingham Palace amid pretty painted porcelain cups and elaborate sterling teapots. Add to the familiarity of this routine with shortbread cookies, scones with sweet jam, or perhaps some finger sandwiches to make afternoon tea a light repast that nourishes both body and spirit.

Recall the exotic feel of Morocco — sit on your living room floor, among heaps of pillows and soft woolen carpets underneath, your host pouring hot steaming mint tea from the narrow pot with the long, long skinny spout into small glasses snuggled into their brass holders.

Conjure up a visit to an esteemed Chinese ceramist. Picture yourself sitting in his lush green garden, listening to

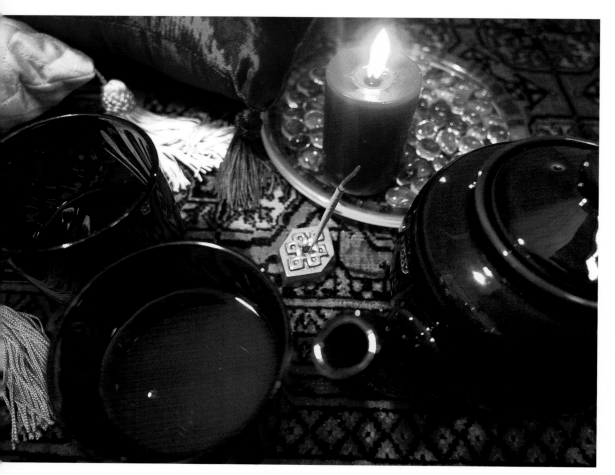

Exotic table accessories and rich fabrics make every visitor for tea feel special, as the caressing scent of incense relaxes all.

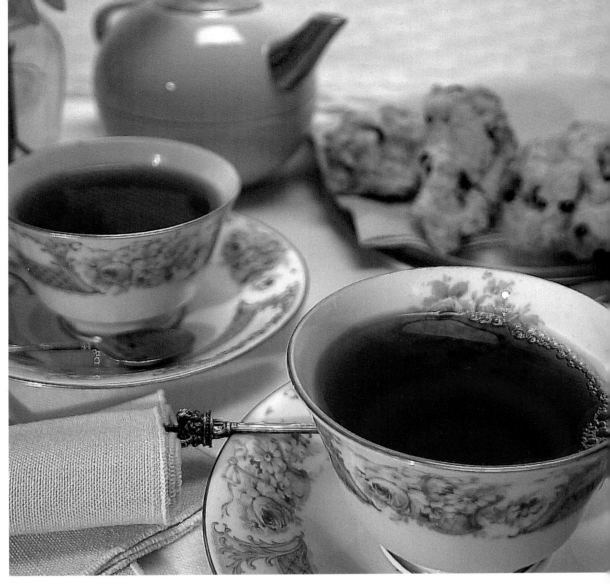

Nothing is more comforting than a familiar round-bellied teapot, yummy scones and other treats, and pretty porcelain cups of steaming tea.

finches overhead, while you drink oolong tea freshly made by his farmer neighbor. Inhale the earthy-sweet perfume of the golden amber liquid as it fills a purple clay cup designed, made, and fired by your host, just for your pleasure.

Perhaps you'd like to tour Japan and partake of its quiet, contemplative ceremony of tea, *chanoyu*. Set the mood right in your own home with silky pillows placed around low tables or a coffee table. Choose a Japanese green tea like sencha or fukimashi-cha and brew it in the customary black iron hobnail teapot, then pour the pale green tea into clear glass or plain white cups to best enjoy the color of the tea. Jean-Pierre Rampal or James Galway playing Japanese favorites on the flute would be the perfect music to transport you to Japan.

The Garden Sanctuary

When I was a child, my family and I moved into the very first home of our own, where we were fortunate to have a wonderful backyard and evergreen trees bordering three sides of the property. The previous owner had planted the trees so close together that they folded into one another at the edge of the property to form a densely shaded, cool, and very intensely green curtain.

In one corner of the backyard, hardly visible through the heavy branches, was a miniature Japanese garden with a small two-foot pond with goldfish, a graceful red bridge stretching from one side of the pond to the other, and a circle of variegated rocks circling the water and giving protection to the fish.

I used to sit by this quiet nook for hours, smelling the unmistakable pungency of pine needles brushing my hair and watching the fish swim around fallen leaves to pursue their daily bread crumbs. At 12 years old, I was unaware of words like serenity, meditation, and centering, yet I received all three as gifts from this jewel-like little oasis of calm. As an adult, I understand better how being among nature can nourish one in so many ways, every day.

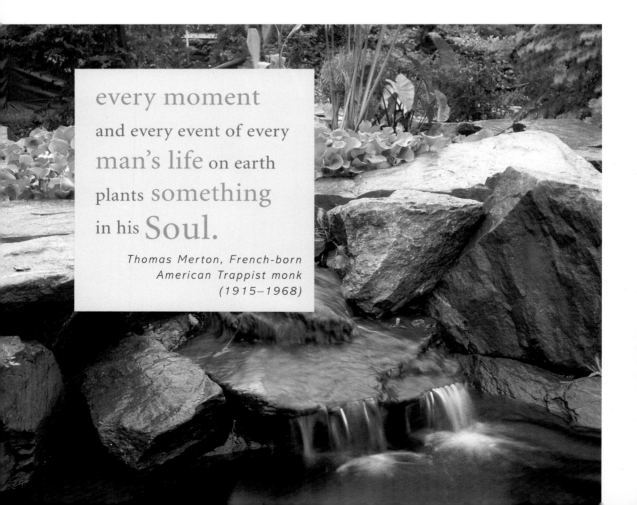

every moment and every event of every man's life on earth plants something in his Soul.

Thomas Merton, French-born
American Trappist monk
(1915–1968)

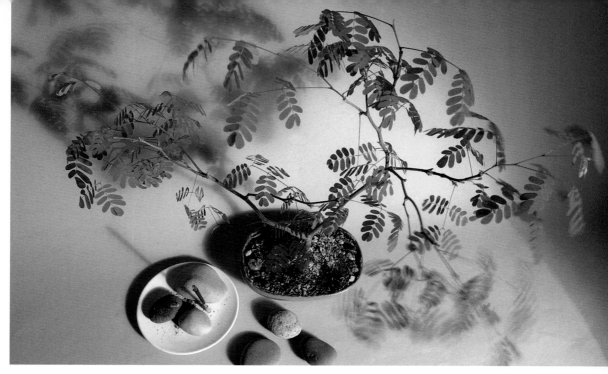

A delicate bonsai tree is a striking reminder
of the beauty of the natural world.

giving back to Nature

If you have a compost pile in your
garden, you can discard the ashes
from your incense burning directly into
the pile. Ash is a good additive to compost, and any leftover fragrance from
the incense certainly couldn't hurt the
aroma of the pile. ✳

Creating a Garden Altar

A garden altar can be without any traditional religious significance but can
reflect, instead, the beauty of nature her-
self. Consider arrangements of treasured
pebbles, a sand garden dotted with
bonsai, a koi pond edged with protective
grasses. Anything that touches your heart
and brings you peace when you look
upon it can be considered a garden altar.

Planting trees or flowers to cherish the
memory of someone you love needs no
altar or labeling; the quiet loveliness of a
rose, the vibrant color of a hibiscus, the
strength of an oak tree — any of these
marvels of nature is altar enough to
remind you of that special someone.

Statuary of Buddha, the Virgin Mary,
or other religious icons can be part of a
garden altar to which you can offer
morning or evening prayers or your own
personal spiritual reflections.

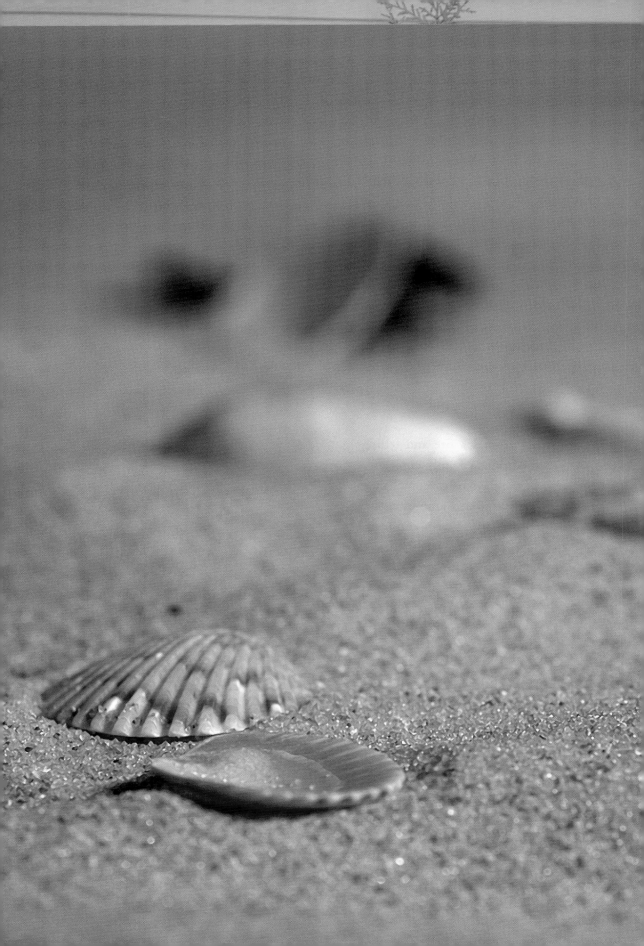

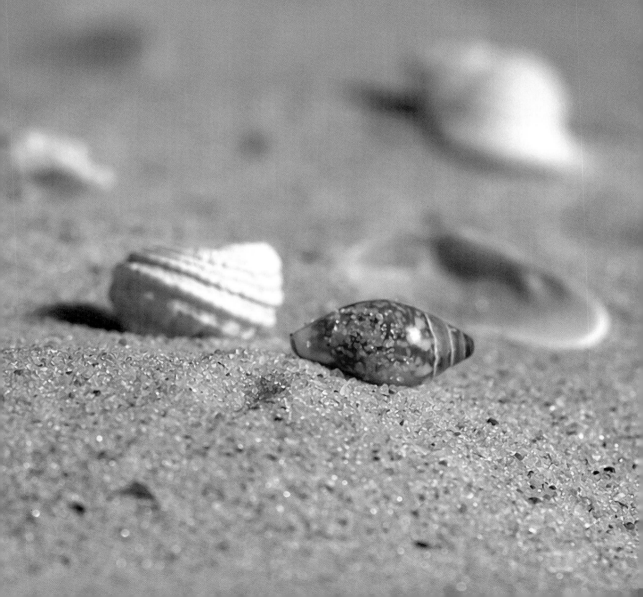

A Perfect End to a Day

Fire invites us to relax in the grace of company. Building a bonfire on a starry summer night at the beach, or kicking back around the woodstove or fireplace after a day of skiing, hiking, or doing chores — a roaring fire offers a wonderful chance to regroup, relax, and bask in the group spirit.

Incense and fire are made for each other. Mix a cone or two into the fire and breathe in the refreshing scent of incense mixed with wood smoke. It will calm you and bring clarity to your mind and a sense of peace to your heart. The warmth of the flame will embrace you while the storytelling begins.

Invoking the
Storytelling Tradition

Women have always gathered together to share tasks, offer friendship, pass on wisdom, and seek and receive advice on mothering and homekeeping. This coming together has produced magnificent quilts from sewing bees, enlightenment from prayer circles, and better knowledge of the intimate details of marriage.

In the Hispanic culture, one such gathering of women is the *tertulia*, a regularly scheduled meeting where women share their joys, expunge their sorrows, eat good food, and provide all the comforts of dynamic and supportive friendships.

Men, too, have gathered together to frame homes, help one another during the harvest, and attach to the spiritual in sweat lodges. They have danced like dervishes, played drums together, or performed less exotic connections to the spiritual by one-on-one mentoring of youth interested in their career fields.

Fortunately, more and more men are sharing feelings and ideas, allowing themselves more dips into the reservoir of their dreams and fears and hopes. The oral tradition of telling fables to teach is as ancient as fire itself and the perfect way to share storytelling experiences with children or teenagers.

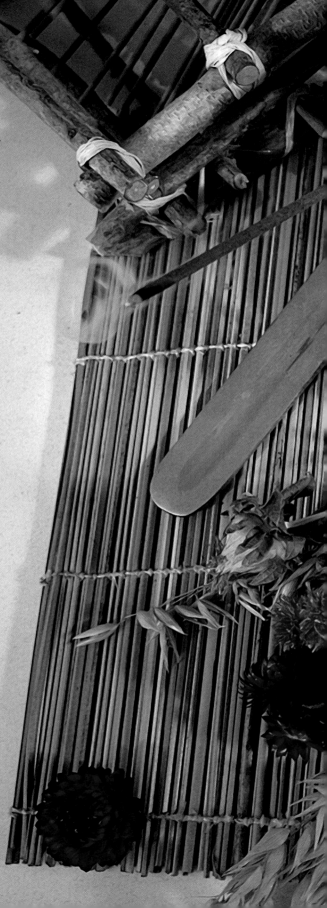

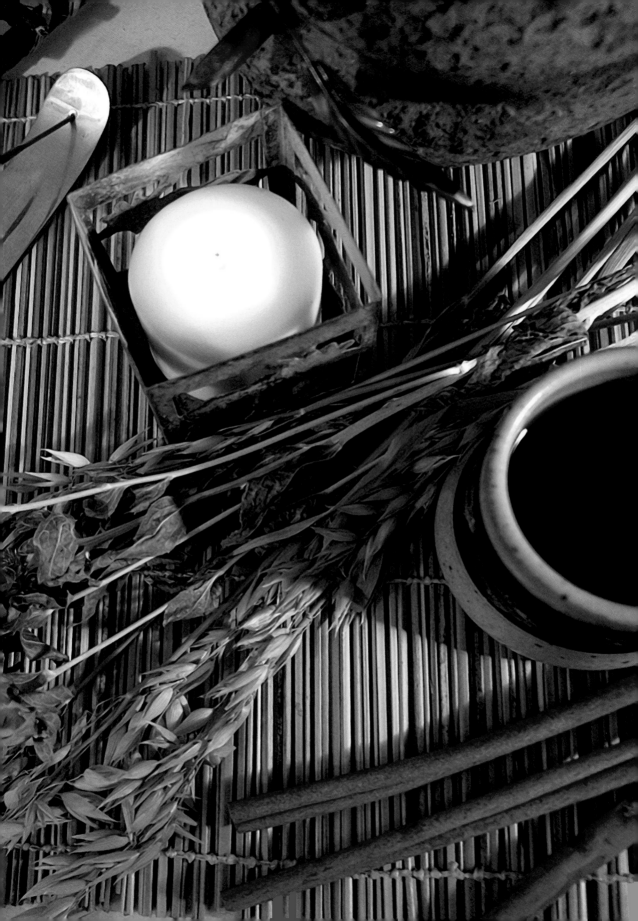

the story of Shingebiss

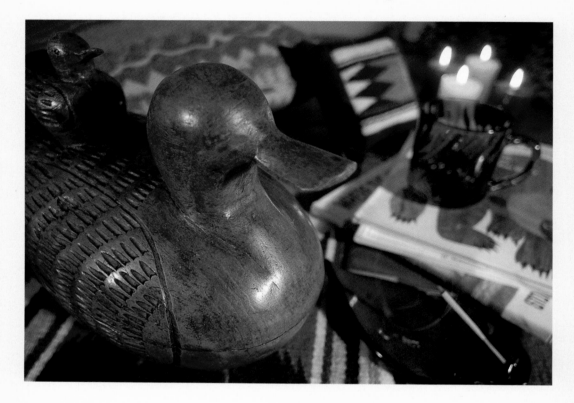

There may be someone in your group who is a natural storyteller, or someone may emerge once the stories start. Traditionally, the storytelling starts with the eldest man or woman in the group, who can choose whatever story to tell. One inspiration is the Bible; fairytales and myths are others. Folk tales that reflect your heritage are particularly vivid examples of the oral tradition, or you may want to recount this classic Chippewa tale about a little brown duck named Shingebiss who well understood his own power.

Along the shores of Lake Huron lived a little brown duck named Shingebiss. Brave and cheery was he, even when the fierce North Wind blew down from the glittering silver Land of Snow. No matter how the North Wind raged, the little brown duck always found food to nourish himself, and great logs for firewood for his little lodge.

He pulled up frozen rushes from the nearby pond, dove down through the holes left by the rushes, and fished for his supper. Pulling a string of fish behind him, he walked leisurely back to his lodge, cooked the fish to perfection on his blazing fire, and made himself warm and cozy.

The North Wind screamed, "Woo-oo-oo! Who dares brave Big Chief North Wind? All of the other creatures fear him. Only Shingebiss ignores me!"

The North Wind sent colder, icier blasts; showered high drifts of snow upon the ground; and soon not one bird nor beast dared venture forth, except for Shingebiss. The little brown duck continued to dive for his fish, gather logs, cook his supper, and warm himself by his fire.

"Arrgh!" cried Big Chief North Wind. "Shingebiss cares not for snow nor ice. I will freeze the holes of his pond so he cannot get fish. I will conquer him."

So the North Wind froze the holes of the ponds wherever the little brown duck fished, and blanketed the ponds with heaping piles of heavy snow.

Shingebiss uttered not one word when he found his fishing holes closed. He cheerfully walked on until he found another pond in which to fish. He pulled up the rushes and made new holes and fished for his supper, and he cut new logs and took them all home, where he ate his fish by the warm and cozy fire in his lodge.

The North Wind howled in anger for days and days and days. Wherever the little brown duck went, the North Wind followed, freezing the holes in the ponds and covering each pond high with snow.

Shingebiss walked farther and farther, fearlessly, as he always had done. And always he found yet another pond in which to fish.

One evening, Big Chief North Wind quietly crept up to the warm and cozy lodge of the little brown duck. Shingebiss could feel the icy cold float through the cracks of the door, yet he sang quietly to himself:

North Wind, North Wind, fierce in feature
You are still my fellow creature
Blow your worst, you can't freeze me
I fear you not, and so I'm FREE!

Big Chief North Wind sat down by little Shingebiss and muttered angrily, "I will freeze you! I will stay until you are frozen!"

Just at that moment, Shingebiss leaned over and stirred his fire. The logs glowed red and gold and a shower of sparks leapt into the air. All at once, the North Wind's frosty hair began to drip; his icy face started to dissolve; and the mighty biting cold puff of his breath grew fainter.

Shingebiss just sat, warming his little webbed feet by the blaze, and kept singing quietly:

North Wind, North Wind, fierce in feature
You are still my fellow creature.

North Wind screamed, "Big Chief is melting!" Rushing headlong through the doorway, he flung himself onto a snowbank, mumbling, "Strange Shingebiss. I cannot starve him. I cannot freeze him. I cannot make him afraid. Ah, North Wind will let Shingebiss alone now, for the Great Spirit is with him."

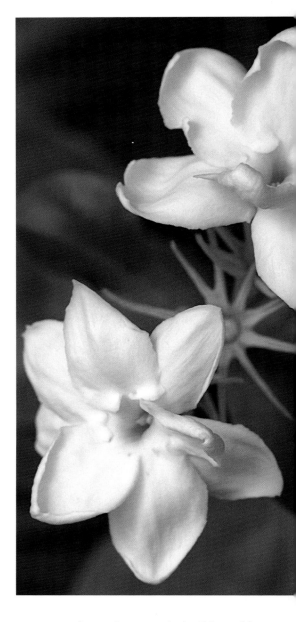

Let mystery have
its place in you;
Do not be always turning
up your whole soil
with the ploughshares of
self-examination,
But leave a little fallow
corner in your heart
Ready for any seed
the winds
may bring.

Henri Frederic Amiel,
Swiss critic (1821–1861)

Jasmine creates a positive state of consciousness that is particularly conducive to journaling. Its sweet, fresh fragrance inspires creativity, creates a soothing atmosphere, and leaves one refreshed and clear in mind and spirit. Jasmine has a light stimulating effect on the eros and works on the second chakra. Thus, if you want to write a love letter or pen a romantic story, jasmine is definitely the incense to choose.

Incense made with Tibetan or Chinese jasmine has a particularly delicate scent. Jasmine is uplifting, balancing, helps with stress and anxiety, and builds self-confidence — even more reason to write about all the things you love. By taking the time to write down all the ideas that may swim in your mind, you are better able to see which ideas to pursue and which to eliminate or postpone. You may even learn new ways to do the ordinary.

The Joys of Journaling

A stationery store to a writer is like a candy store to a child: All the possibilities! Today, the choices are nearly infinite, from vellums to watermarked sheets and handmade leaf-embedded papers in every color of the rainbow.

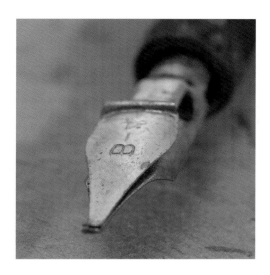

As inviting as papers are, pens can be even more tempting, for they are tools of expression and style. What will you choose? A smooth rollerball, or that Venetian glass quill and inkwell? Will it be an antique fountain pen filled with lavender-scented ink, or your trusty #2 lead pencil with graying pink eraser?

The objective, of course, is not to have the prettiest notebook or the most elegant pen, but to use these media of pen and paper to put thoughts down and watch your dreams come alive.

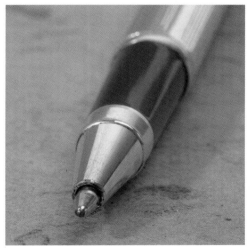

A journal corner should be as private and as beautiful as possible. Adjust the lighting with lamps or natural light from windows, select just the right chair or totally relax by stretching out on a lounge chair or a bed. When you make your body comfortable, your mind can relax quicker and more easily.

Journaling can be a love letter to yourself, an instrument of confidence-building, a method of clearing the mind and finding out who you really are. Journaling is a self-embracing act.

For your personal journal, choose whatever instrument most directly expresses your style.

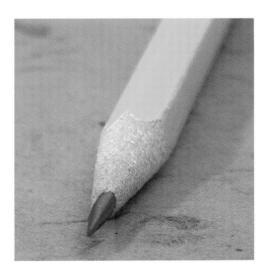

nudging the Muse

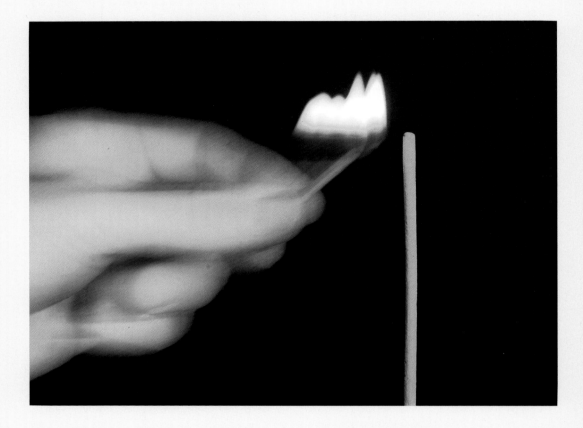

On a bench or a table, set up your accoutrements for lighting your incense. As you strike the match, think about the topics you want to explore. No one but you can enter your thoughts, so go where you need to go. In your own way, ask for guidance or inspiration for what you're about to do.

When the incense begins to smolder, start moving the pen over the pages of your journal. At any pause in your writing, close your eyes and allow the incense to caress you;

inhale its sweetness; daydream. Slowly open your eyes and continue writing without stopping for editing or self-criticism.

Should you be unfamiliar with journal or diary writing, consider using any or all of the following as "warm-ups": Write about your day; write an observation about the natural world or what you see out your window; write a letter to a parent or child; write a poem to your beloved; write about a memorable event; or write down questions

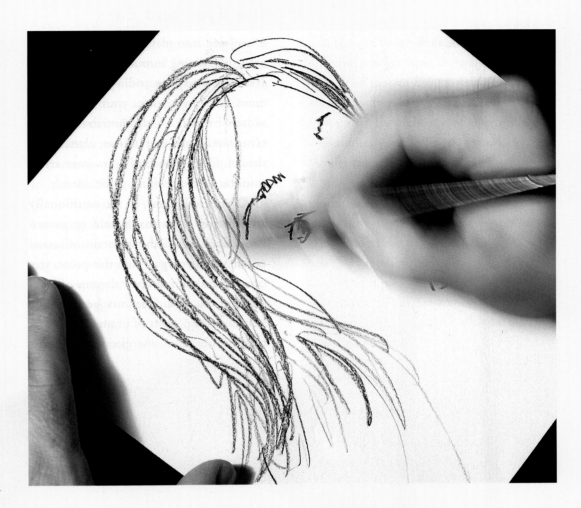

for which you believe you have no answers at the moment.

If drawing is your medium, draw what you see or what you feel, or even make a sketch of how you would like things or people to be. This is the time for pure fantasy, so let your hand fly over the pages with pencil or brush. A journal that combines writing and drawing may be the best way to tap into all sides of your creativity and to fully express what you feel.

Empty your brain of preconceived notions and let your subconscious rise up. Journaling is a method for capturing these deeper thoughts and answering troubling questions you may be reluctant to consider.

Sit still for a few moments more, eyes closed, and express your gratitude for this very special time. Give thanks in your own words, or simply say, "Thank you for the gift of journaling, for this treasured time, for this opportunity to learn."

Traditional aloeswood is now available as an import from several Asian countries. It is well worth seeking out, as its delicacy and subtlety cannot be truly duplicated by any other wood. The white flowers of the aloeswood tree emit a sweet, lingering fragrance, though it is actually a fungus in the wood that produces the aromatic resin. Native to northern India, Laos, Cambodia, Malaysia, Indonesia, and Vietnam, aloeswood is called *jin-koh* or *kyana* (a more costly version) in Japanese, *chen xiang* in Chinese, and *agaru* or *tagara* in Sanskrit. Other common names in English are agarwood and oud.

Should you wish to try other woods, choose fruitwoods such as cherry, apple, or pear, or perhaps a maple variety or East Indian sandalwood. You will need only small bits of wood, so carve off as much as you need and save the rest for other Koh-Doh experiences.

If you want to use stick incense instead, simply place commercial sticks of incense in the censer filled with white ash, rather than following the more traditional (and more complex) way of Koh-Doh described on pages 104 and 105.

Sweetly aromatic woods connect you to the centuries—old Japanese way of incense.

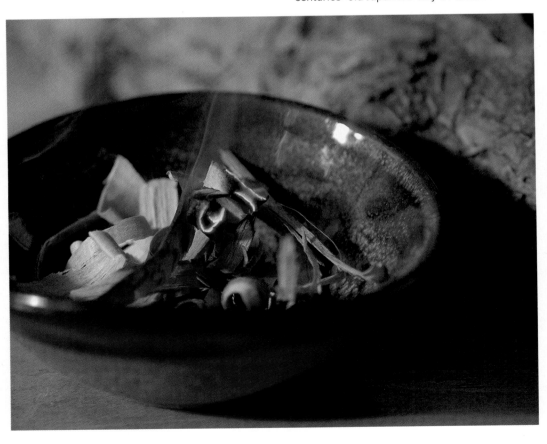

the legend of Aloeswood

Legend has it that centuries ago there washed up upon the shore of Awaji, an island off Japan, a piece of wood unknown to the natives. They let it dry, and when it was ready, they tossed it upon the campfire to help cook their food and warm their families. As the mysterious wood burned, a pleasing aroma echoed upward, mesmerizing the community. One of the leaders pulled out the fragrant wood and extinguished the fire.

For many years after this, whenever it was necessary to appease the gods, the leaders carved out a bit from this solitary piece of wood, burned it, and offered its remarkable smoke as food for the spirits. This aged fragrant wood is now known as aloeswood. ✳

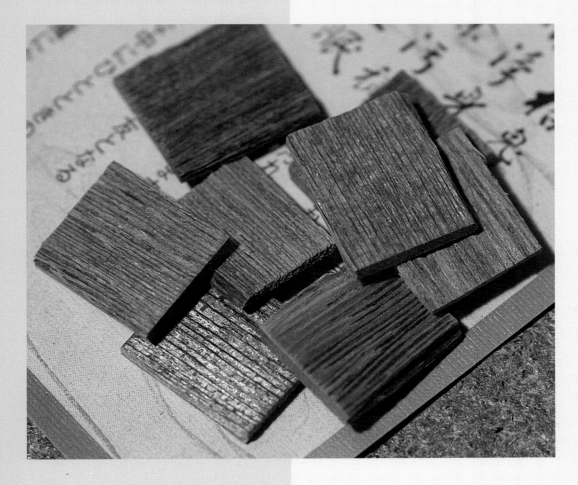

The Koh-Doh Ceremony

Although you can purchase a complete set of Koh-Doh accessories from any fine Japanese incense manufacturer (see Sources on page 121), you may already have most of the needed items around your house. An exception is the white rice ash, which is available at most shops that sell incense products or Asian gifts. If you can't find the ash, ordinary sand or soil can be substituted.

> No one spoke,
>
> The host, the guest,
>
> The white chrysanthemums.
>
> *Oshima Ryota, Japanese poet*
> *(1718–1787)*

Koh-Doh Accessories

- Porcelain Koh-Doh cup to use as a censer (or any small fireproof heavy porcelain bowl)
- Charcoal for incense (do *not* use charcoal briquettes, but only the charcoal expressly made for incense, available at incense suppliers or Catholic gift shops)
- White rice ash, or sand
- Flat knife, to use as an ash press
- Metal chopstick or skewer, to handle hot charcoal
- Piece of mica
- One small piece of aloeswood or other aged aromatic wood
- Metal tweezers

Koh-Doh requires a censer, charcoal, sand or ash, mica, a fragrant wood, and a few easily available tools.

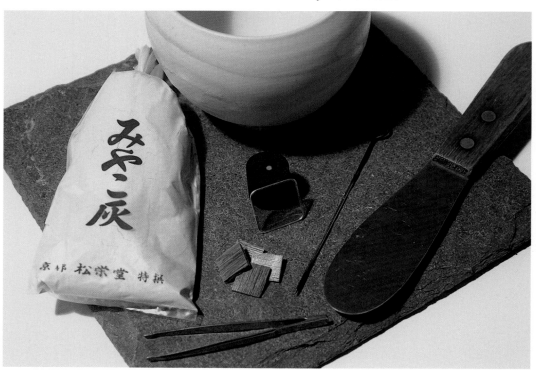

Starting the Incense

1 Fill the Koh-Doh cup about two-thirds full with white rice ash or sand, packing it down firmly.

2 Light a piece of charcoal in a fireproof bowl and heat it until it is grayish-white all over.

3 Using the flat knife or ash press, loosen and fluff up the ash.

4 Using a metal tweezer or tongs, place charcoal on top of the ash in the center of the cup, pushing it about halfway down into the cup. **Do not touch the charcoal with your fingers!**

5 Cover the charcoal completely with the ash until a soft mound forms on top of it.

6 Using the knife again, lightly tamp the ash covering the charcoal into a cone or pyramid shape.

7 With a metal chopstick or skewer, make a small hole through the ash and into the charcoal to allow the air to pass through so the incense will continue to burn.

8 Using the tweezers or tongs, place the mica plate gently on top of the air hole and press softly until it rests flat.

9 Finally, place your piece of aloeswood on top of the mica plate.

10 Sit back and "listen to the incense."

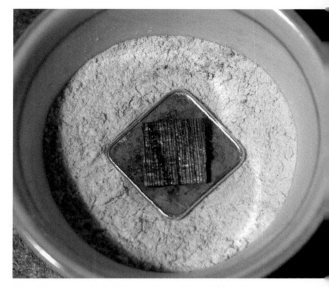

An aloeswood chip rests on mica and burning charcoal to release its essence.

easing Grief

Nearly every religion has embraced aloeswood in its incense ceremonies. Both myrrh and aloeswood were used at the burial of Jesus. The Japanese anoint the dead with aloeswood. The Sufis include oil of aloeswood in their religious rituals, famous for whirling dancing routines that last for hours. Because of its alleged psychoactive properties, aloeswood is often used to treat exhaustion, alleviate neurosis or obsessive behavior, and to ease grief, just as frankincense has been used for centuries. ✳

playful Enjoyment

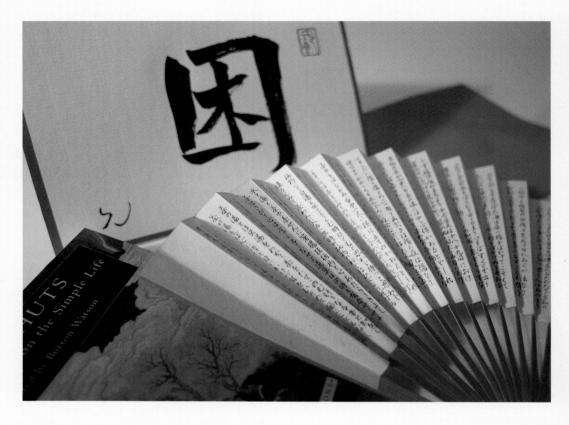

The Japanese are often playful during Koh-Doh, the incense ceremony. Invite the fragrance of incense to inspire your sense of play by simply lighting a stick of Japanese incense to scent the room while you're playing word games like Pictionary or Scrabble, cards, or favorite board games. Japanese incense is much subtler and more delicate than East Indian or most commercial incense and will be less intrusive while, at the same time, it creates the relaxing mood you want for this exercise.

Concentrating on the games, relaxing in the pleasant incense, and avoiding the cacophony of radio and television and life's other noises will bring you great peace and a lot of sweet joy from the simplicity of playing together.

If you want to match the more literary style of Koh-Doh, you can write haiku, the unusual Japanese poem that has 17 syllables divided into three lines of five, seven, and five syllables each. Some slight variations to this syllable count result when haikus are translated into English.

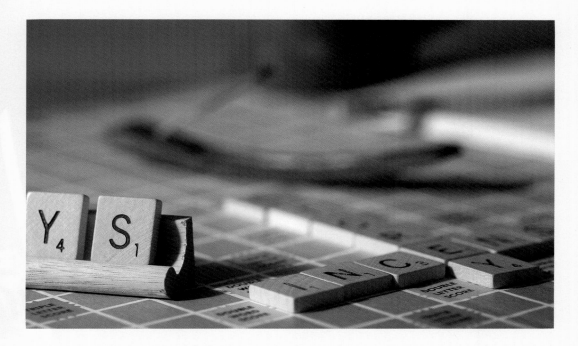

Here is a classic example from the Japanese poet Taniguchi Buson, also known as Yosa Buson (1716–1783):

Over vast fields of mustard
Moon rises eastward
Sun sets in the west.

And here are two haiku from the poet Kobayashi Issa (1763–1827):

In my life as in
The twilight, bells sound
The freshness of evening.

Wild goose, wild goose, tell me, at
what age did you fly
on your first journey?

For a theme for your own poem, consider the seasons and their colors, one of the most popular haiku topics. Light another incense stick for inspiration. Perhaps a delicate lotus, sensuous ylang-ylang, or Kashmir rose will offer just the right atmosphere for creativity.

Or, why not consider writing a group poem? Write one line on a piece of paper, and hand it to the person beside you, folding the paper down so that each subsequent person sees only the line written by her neighbor. She will write down the second line, then pass it on to the third person, who will add a third line, and so forth around the room. The result? Either a hilarious or a remarkably wonderful poem. These collaborative works, which are known as *renga,* are another spin on Japanese poetry and are always great fun.

Here are some suggested first lines to get your communal poem started:

Viewing the snow-capped mountain, I . . .
Birds chirping in the air . . .
The trickle of the brook, the brush of a breeze
*   through the trees . . .*

Spring is also a time to refresh and reawaken our homes after the dormancy of winter living. In the past, spring cleaning was an elaborate and very effective custom to clean away the heaviness of winter living, to clear away the dust of hibernation, to welcome the birth of spring. If you've fallen away from this tradition, perhaps you can incorporate the ritual into your life once more.

This year, do your own version of spring cleaning. Rid your rooms of clutter. Give away clothes you haven't worn in years. Discard tools and knick-knacks you never use. Ask your children to participate, to give away toys they've tired of or outgrown. Ask your mate to pack at least two boxes of things to clear out of the house for good. Load everything into the car to donate to the charitable organization of your choice.

Rather have a tag sale? Go for it, but promise yourself that anything left over leaves the house for good!

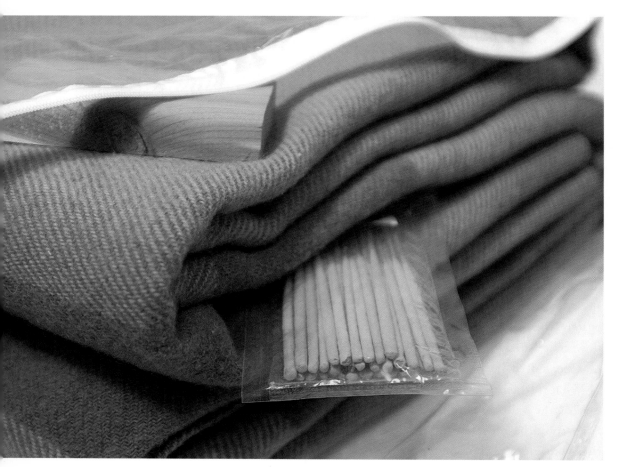

When packing away your winter blankets, add cedar-infused incense sticks or pinion incense cones for an unusual twist on tradition.

Now you're ready to clean! Gather up rugs and air them outdoors; remove paintings and wash down walls; rent or purchase a cleaner to freshen upholstered furnishings and carpets, and to polish floors. Change from heavy blankets and comforters to lightweight bedding. Store winter clothes, adding cedar cones, chips, or incense in packages to keep the moths away.

This ritual of spring cleaning is not only about ridding the house of the old, the dated, the unwanted, but, more important, about ridding yourself of old behaviors. Perhaps you can mark the season by breaking old habits, trying new styles of dress or hair, making new friends, seeking out new experiences, and, most important, remembering to celebrate the renewal of your life with grace and gratitude. You might:

- Celebrate spring by bringing flowers inside to decorate your home.

- Buy a wild and wacky hat.

- Break away from routines: Go for walks in the park; take up tennis again; sign up for a new sport at the Y.

- Gather your family around you to bless your fresh-as-spring home. Light incense with the freshest, most energizing citrus scents you can find: mandarin, grapefruit, lime — whatever pleases you.

- Offer your gratitude and love for one another, and the blessing of a home freshly clean, safe, and in peace.

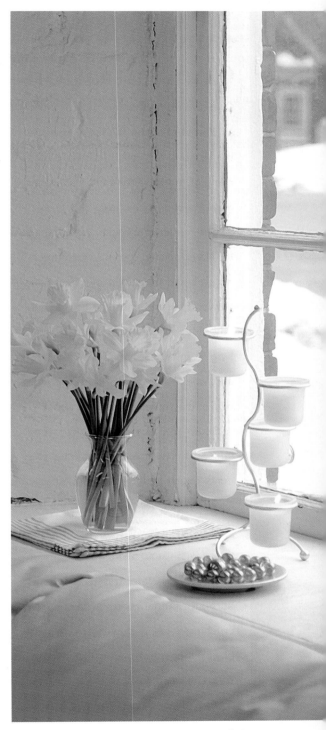

Buttery yellow daffodils are a perfect gift for your home after a vigorous spring cleaning.

Fall Comforts

Browns, golds, yellows, oranges, and dark reds color the season of fall as leaves change on trees, pumpkins and other favorite squash are harvested, and foods take on the spices of the season.

These seasonings are exceptionally wonderful choices as scents for spicy, invigorating incense to mark this new season in your personal or home rituals. Some of the scents that you might want to try are mixtures of allspice, orange blossoms, and any of the earthy, woodsy fragrances such as frankincense, myrrh, cedar, and pine.

These aromas spell fall in all its aspects. You can now pick your harvest from the bounty you planted during the summer. Share it with fellow gardeners over for a "surplus swap," trading your plethora of zucchini for someone else's abundance of tomatoes and another's extra chives.

Select a little of the harvest from everyone present and make a gigantic pot of vegetable soup with plenty to fill containers or bowls to be taken home later. Bake or buy the freshest bread that you can, and dine in splendor on a genuinely communal meal. Could anything be more wonderful than a meal made from the bounty of everyone's garden?

Scents
of the season

With the bounty of the harvest available, autumn is a perfect time for creating your own natural incense. Capturing the feeling of fall with incense is as easy as pie: Choose classic spices such as sage, clove, or allspice. Or light two different sources of incense, perhaps one spice variety and one refreshing citrus scent to recall favorite scent memories. ✳

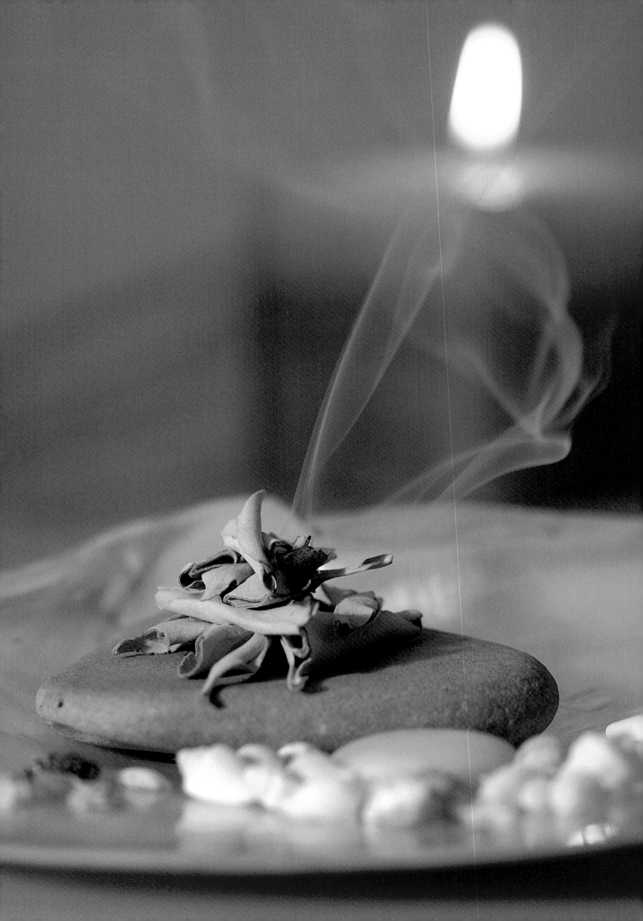

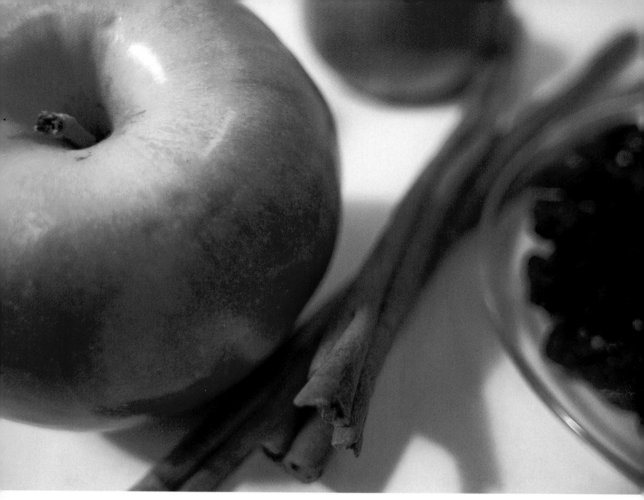

What smells like fall? Baked apples and cinnamon? Autumn is as near as your incense burner.

Fall is a rewarding time to enjoy the fruits of your garden, to join together more often with friends at home, and to prepare for the quiet restorative season of winter. Perhaps you'll want to enroll in cooking classes, update your family tree project, or plan that midwinter vacation to someplace exotic and warm! Or you could:

- Make sauce from extra tomatoes and more veggie soup; freeze them for later.

- Prepare for winter by checking out the heater and the fireplace now, before the first chill. Bring out the winter clothes and the winter bedding. Consider donating extra blankets and outgrown winter clothes to shelters for the homeless.

- Go back to school to learn something that you've always wanted to: playing the piano, tango dancing, painting murals, how to tune up your car, a new language — whatever intrigues or delights you.

- Make s'mores.

- Make every day Thanksgiving by remembering your bounty of food, shelter, friends, and family.

Winter Slumbers

In some places, winter is so cold, you'll wonder if your sense of smell will freeze as much as the radiator in your car. In other places, winter is simply cooler, brisker, with only some bare trees to signal the change of season.

As nature slumbers, we slow ourselves down during the winter months. The fragrance of a winter fire of scented woods is a peaceful way to end a day. Cedar, pine, pinion, and the scents of the table like orange, cinnamon, and clove, all invite a sense of warmth with their comforting, familiar aromas.

Now is the time to focus on one another instead of the world outside, to pop corn and watch your favorite videos, eat hot pizzas with hot cocoa even on school nights, and enjoy the beauty of your home and the joy of your friends and family.

This is not to suggest doing nothing. You could:

- Get brochures now to plan your summer vacation. Look at the videotapes or photos from last year's explorations. Make a scrapbook.

- Tell stories to one another in front of the fire or amid the warmth of a kitchen while baking cookies or roasting chestnuts.

- Write letters the old-fashioned way, on beautiful stationery with elegant pen and ink.

- Reread favorite books or do a twist on the book club theme: Have a "book swap." Each participant brings two books. (This is great for children, too, to trade for other books.) After each donor reveals why his two books were great reads, he can take two "new" books home to read over the winter. While swapping books, drink hot chocolate or hot masala chai.

- Light up a cone of frankincense, the fragrance of peace, as you enter the new year. Recall memories of the past year and think of ways to celebrate or honor the seasons in even more vital and life-affirming ways. Offer gratitude once more for friendships, health, enough to share, for the opportunity to begin anew.

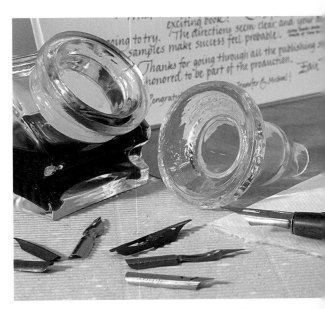

A cold winter night is the perfect time to write a special letter to a friend you see too rarely.

appendix: how to make incense

Perhaps the easiest way to make incense at home is to place naturally dried herbs in a fireproof bowl and light them with a match. Extinguish the flame, fan the end with your hand or a feather, and allow the incense to burn. Sage, cedar chips, even dried cassia and cloves work well.

For incense sticks, buying them ready-made is simpler and often even less expensive than making your own. Still, there are several wonderful reasons for making incense by hand: You can choose any fragrance or combination of fragrances, form it into any shape or size you want, and expand this into a very satisfying hobby. Handmade incense is a delightfully different and appealing gift.

The Main Ingredients

The following are the most common ingredients for handmade incense. They can be found at most shops or online resources that carry incense, or at a chemical supply shop or a pharmacy.

Essential oils, or incense oils, are pure essences of plants and flowers. One to three drops will usually be more than enough. NEVER use synthetic oils or perfume oils, because they are toxic when burned.

Resins are the sticky residue from plants or trees used for binding the ingredients together in incense. The most popular varieties of resins come from trees, such as sandalwood, camphor, pine, eucalyptus, aloeswood, and cedar. Fossil resins like Russian or Bombay amber are also common.

Gum arabic is the resinous sap that seeps out from the dried gray bark of trees of the genus *Acacia,* especially *A. Senegal.* Benzoin is a resin known for its vanilla-like aroma and its efficacy as a binding ingredient in incense.

Basic Safety Rules

Safety measures to follow when making incense include:

• Always wear gloves.

• Always prepare incense in a well-ventilated room.

• Always keep everything away from children and pets.

• Buy incense ingredients from reputable chemists, pharmacists, or incense suppliers you trust. Whenever possible, choose raw materials over "natural" ones that may contain some toxic binders or fillers.

• Allow five to seven days for the incense to dry thoroughly.

• If using saltpeter, *never* use more than 10 percent of it for the entire combination of ingredients. If less than 10 percent is added, the incense may not ignite; if too much is added, the incense will ignite too quickly and may explode.

Basic Equipment

If at all possible, all equipment and tools, especially the measuring spoons, mortar and pestle or grinder, should be dedicated to incense making. Glass bowls are preferable, because they can be cleaned thoroughly, though they also should not be used for other purposes. Necessary equipment includes:

• Latex gloves
• Mortar and pestle or grinder
• One set of measuring spoons
• One large and two small glass bowls
• One cotton or linen washcloth, dampened with hot water
• One medicine dropper (for the essential oils)
• Kitchen scale (cover with wax paper if also used for food)
• 10 to 30 bamboo skewers
• Large block of Styrofoam
• 6 to 12 plastic bags large enough to store the incense you plan to make

Note: A spice or coffee grinder works well but should be dedicated to incense making only. Mixing the spices for incense with food spices will contaminate the food and possibly make you ill.

Basic Ingredients List

8 ounces of warm water
1 teaspoon of gum arabic (tragacanth can be used instead, but will require slightly more water)
2 tablespoons ground benzoin
1 tablespoon ground orrisroot
8 tablespoons sandalwood powder, divided
4 to 9 drops lemon or other essential oil
1 1/2 tablespoons myrrh powder
1/2 tablespoon eucalyptus powder
1 to 3 ounces saltpeter (potassium nitrate), depending upon total amount of incense made

Note: If possible, buy powdered ingredients preground, as grinding can take hours. Otherwise, grind the orrisroot, sandalwood, eucalyptus, and other fragrances with a mortar and pestle until a fine powder results.

Making Incense Sticks

1 In a small glass bowl, combine gum arabic and warm water until it forms a thick paste. Add a little more water as necessary. It should look like thick, gooey oatmeal. Cover the bowl with a hot dampened cloth and set it aside.

2 In a large glass bowl, mix together the benzoin, orrisroot, and 6 tablespoons of the sandalwood. Add 3 to 6 drops of essential oil, using the eyedropper. Mix thoroughly with latex-gloved hands. In another small bowl, mix the myrrh, eucalyptus, and 2 tablespoons sandalwood. This mixture should appear powdery yet fine grained. Add 1 to 3 drops of essential oil to bind the powders.

3 Weigh the mixture from the large bowl on the scale. Measure out enough saltpeter to equal 10 percent of its weight. For example, for 10 ounces of incense, add one ounce of saltpeter and mix thoroughly.

4 Remove cloth from bowl of gum arabic paste. To test the paste, dip a skewer into it. The mixture should be thin enough for the skewer to dip into it yet thick enough that the stick can stand in it without falling over. If it is not thick enough, mix in more gum arabic.

5 Add the paste to the large-bowl mixture a little at a time, just until the powdered ingredients are thoroughly dampened.

6 Dip about one-third to one-half of the skewer surface into this paste. Then dip the skewer into the powdery ingredients from the small bowl. You may need to do this several times until enough fragrance attaches itself to the stick (about ⅛ inch thick). Allow each layer of powdered fragrance ingredients to dry thoroughly (three to five minutes or longer) before adding the next layer.

7 Stick the bare ends of the skewers into a Styrofoam block to dry. When all the skewers are covered and placed upright in the Styrofoam, set them aside in a warm, dry, well-ventilated place for five to seven days. If they do not dry completely, they will not ignite.

8 When completely dry, store incense sticks in heavy polyurethane bags large enough to cover them without crushing.

Making Cone Incense

For cones, you will need the all the above equipment and ingredients, except for the Styrofoam and the skewers. You will also need wax paper and some cone forms, available from baking and cooking supply shops.

1 In a small glass bowl, combine the gum arabic with warm water until it forms a very thick paste, like moist dough. Cover the bowl with a hot dampened cloth and set aside.

2 and 3 Follow steps 2 and 3 on page 119.

4 Wearing latex gloves, place mixture on wax paper and shape into cones, either free form or using 1½- or 1¾-inch bakery cones or a cookie cutter.

5 Set the cones upright on the waxed paper and allow to dry in a well-ventilated dry area for three to seven days. Wearing latex gloves, gently turn them each day to ensure uniform drying without cracking. They will shrink slightly.

6 Store cones in small plastic bags or glass jars and place them in a cool dark cupboard.

resources

Adventure Arabia
Tel: 011 44 1202 462021; fax: 011 44 20 7681 3614
www.adventurearabia.com
This British company imports classic frankincense and myrrh and incense oils directly from the primary growing region in Oman.

Anna's Incense
(604) 869-2796; fax (604) 869-3683
www.annasincense.com
E-mail: info@annasincense.com
Offers a wide selection of fresh incense sticks, cones and coils, incense oils, burners, and fresh-packed sage.

Avid Inc.
P.O. Box 903
New Paltz, NY 12561
(800) 811-2843
E-mail: info@avidgift.com
Incense, incense holders, and other gift products.

Baieido
www.baieido.com
The premier Japanese incense maker since 1657. Uses all-natural, delicately scented ingredients in a wide variety of styles including coils, cones, and sticks.

Blue Pearl Incense
(877) 890-6336
www.bluepearl.com
E-mail: info@bluepearlincense.com
Sells a variety of resins, oils, and traditional incense

Katmandu Incense & Imports
(800) 282-4982; fax (407) 971-2308
www.incense.twoffice.com
E-mail: cleduc@mpinet.net
Sells frankincense and myrrh.

Capricorns Lair
(801) 334-9442; fax (801) 334-9443
www.capricornslair.com
Elegant burners, handmade neri-koh balls, ash, aloeswood chips, and a wide selection of classic incense and supplies for making incense yourself.

Fox Hollow Farm
(888) 371-7627 or (831) 637-4858
www.foxhollowherbs.com
Excellent bundles of sage, lavender and sweetgrass are grown and dried by this family business.

International Treasure Chest, Inc.
(888) 891-7788 or (215) 702-8691
www.intltreasurechest.com
E-mail: itc@intltreasurechest.com
A selection of frankincense and other traditional incense along with gift accessories.

Le Mélange Home Fragrances
(800) 467-0582
www.lemelange.com
Carries the charming line of Azenta stone burners and scented powders to make your own incense in a variety of fun shapes.

Paula Walla Imports
(860) 490-4258
www.paulawalla.com
Selection of coils, Malaysian and Japanese incense, and Palo Santo aromatic wood from the Amazon.

Pictish Vision
(541) 686-6136
www.celtic.net/pictish
E-mail: pictish@celtic.net
Loose incense formulated to evoke the spirits of the ancient Celts. Requires charcoal tablets to burn.

Shoyeido Incense
(800) 786-5476; fax (888) 435-0005
www.shoyeido.com
E-mail: support @shoyeido.com
A leading Japanese incense producer.

Fred Soll's Natural Incense & Etc.
(505) 889-2924; fax (505) 889-2948
www.fredsoll.com
Offers natural resins and essences, sticks designed to burn horizontally, polymer clay burners guaranteed not to crack, and incense sticks and cones.

Tibetan Incense Company
(435) 644-8749
www.tibetanincense.com
Pure and natural incense following recipes of ancient traditions. Offers Himalayan rope incense, too.

The following brands of Native American bundles and East Indian incense sticks are available at health food stores and incense shops in a variety of fragrances:
Airsworld; Aurshikha; Medicine Wheels Nature Spirits; Nag Champa (Satya Sai Baba); Tra Incense; Triloka

index

other storey titles you will enjoy

The Aromatherapy Companion, by Victoria H. Edwards. The most comprehensive aromatherapy guide available includes profiles of essential oils, instructions for blending and using them, and information on careers in aromatherapy. 288 pages. Paperback. ISBN 1-58017-150-8.

365 Ways to Relax Mind, Body & Soul, by Barbara L. Heller. From simple uplifting thoughts to invigorating exercises, feel-good foods, and diet advice, this book provides hundreds of tips to help you come alive and feel your best day in and day out. 384 pages. Paperback. ISBN 1-58017-332-2.

Feng Shui Dos & Taboos, by Angi Ma Wong. In a fun, A-Z format, the author delivers more than 350 tips, practices, principles, proverbs of feng shui with a focus on the simple and the practical. 416 pages. Paperback. ISBN 1-58017-308-X.

The Handmade Candle, by Alison Jenkins. Includes clear and simple instructions for making designer candles at home for a fraction of the retail cost. 80 pages. Hardcover. ISBN 1-58017-353-5.

Taking Time for Tea, by Diana Rosen. Fabulous menus, recipes, and suggestions for relaxing and celebrating common life experiences over a specially selected cup of tea. 80 pages. Hardcover. ISBN 1-58017-245-8.

The Healing Aromatherapy Bath, by Margo Valentine Lazzara, C.Ht. Combining aromatherapy with hypnotherapy, this hands-on approach to mind/body healing offers 12 essential-oil formulas to be used in the bath in combination with imagery and meditation exercises. 160 pages. Paperback. ISBN 1-58017-197-4.

Making Aromatherapy Creams & Lotions, by Donna Maria. A guide to creating exciting, unique, and personal aromatherapy cosmetics and body-care products from all-natural ingredients. 168 pages. Paperback. ISBN 1-58017-241-5.

Keeping Life Simple, by Karen Levine. This fun, friendly book includes seven guiding principles and hundreds of useful ideas on how to simplify and organize your home, housekeeping, finances, and even your kids. 160 pages. Paperback. ISBN 0-88266-943-5.

Making Herbal Dream Pillows, by Jim Long. Instructions for creating a variety of fragrant dream pillows designed to summon up long-hidden memories and inspire the dreams that you wish for. 64 pages. Paperback. ISBN 1-58017-075-7.

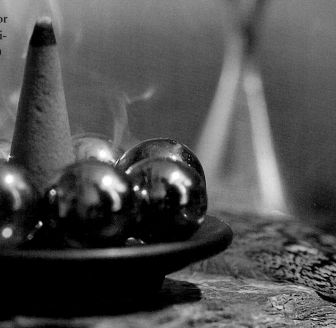